Don Lemmon's
KNOW
HOW:

The TRUTH About
Exercise & Nutrition

BOOK ONE

Written and Copyrighted 1992 – 2002
by Donald E. Lemmon, Jr.

Don Lemmon's KNOW HOW:
The TRUTH About Exercise & Nutrition • BOOK ONE

Written and Copyrighted 1992 – 2002
by Donald E. Lemmon, Jr.
Reviewed by John Ozanich

THE ONLY INTERNATIONALLY RECOGNIZED HEALTH & FITNESS PROGRAM WHERE THE AUTHOR HIMSELF PERSONALLY WELCOMES YOUR E-MAILS!

Kiss your digestive 'dis'-orders and body fat good-bye!

Today's Date Is:
_____ / _____ / _____ (month/day/year)

My Goals Will Be Reached On:
_____ / _____ / _____ (month/day/year)

IN CASE OF LOSS PLEASE NOTIFY:

Name: _____

Street Address: _____

City, State/Province, Postal Code: _____

Country: _____

E-mail Address: _____

Signature: _____

Don Lemmon's FREE Online News Magazine:
http://www.yougottareadthis.com

For Program Questions Contact:
editor@yougottareadthis.com

"Nothing is as efficient as ALLOWING the body to do what it does naturally. The only way to succeed is to pay attention to the natural laws of human chemistry. My objective is met by providing you with an education system that not only stimulates rapid results, but followed as outlined, should command the interest of every physician who claims to follow a preventative health care philosophy."

This book is a compilation of all other editions coming before it. Anything missing from other editions was found to be redundant but a lot of this book has been updated and improved upon. This book was also again not professionally edited because we didn't feel it needed an editor. I prefer to write like I speak, right off the top of my head. I wanted you to know what I was thinking as opposed to someone else's interpretation thereof.

I am not perfect. I am not a professional writer. Odds are you aren't a pro either. If you go into this as a supplemental educational tool, you're going to come out shining. I am a simple nutrition consultant who spent the first half of his professional career as an exercise advisor. Bear with my mistakes and grammatical errors.

The original transcript for this manual was written over a weekend and each revision was done in day's time as well. I do not know many other people that have sat down and rattled off what they knew so quickly and ended up with so much usable information as I am presenting, so please, just take things for what they are worth. Not what you think would have been your approach instead.

While the book is not professionally edited, several hardheaded, grumpy old physicians who made suggestions to ensure a sound presentation have over the years, reviewed it. In other words, before you write off what I do as ridiculous, I can assure you, it's sound.

No part of this publication shall be misconstrued, reproduced in any way, shape, or form whatsoever without prior permission in writing. You DON'T want to make my attorney testy so do not make illegal copies or quote me in print without being granted permission first. Trust me on this. We do not tolerate thieves.

By bending, folding, tearing or marking in this book with pen or pencil, you have voided the ability to receive a refund. I worked very hard to complete this project. You paid a fee to own it and have contact with me for 30 days in doing so. Dr. Atkins, Barry Sears, Tony Little, Suzanne Somers, Richard Simmons and Bill Phillips do not offer that much. Since each purchase is registered to one and only one user each, please simply refer your friends and family to pick up a copy of their own if they want counseling too. That isn't too much to ask. Besides, we need all the additional business we can get just to support my Chihuahua's insatiable steak and chicken diet. Are these animals supposed to eat their weight in meat and not gain an ounce? Whoa.

I thank those who supported my efforts and allowing me to hide away from the World to create this product and my supplement line. I appreciate the unconditional love and support so many have given over the years. It is said a person's life is a reflection of the support they receive. I believe we are what we are and do what we do because of the decisions we make in life. May this book reflect the support I received and the decisions I have made completely.

Once you're done reading, feel free to drop me a line. Do not forget to let me know if you want to begin or continue to receive our monthly supplement club refills after your initial order. We re-ship to you every 30 days and you may cancel at anytime prior to each delivery. You may also request we ship every 5, 6 or 9 weeks if you prefer.

In regards to the supplements or this book, we know you'll enjoy, so please do...

ISBN# 0-9713602-1-9

Published in the United States by the Don Lemmon Company.
Printed in Quebec, Canada

Cover & Book Design: Jason Gateman of www.thinkbigdesigns.com

1st Printing – Burbank, California June 1992
2nd Printing – Boardman, Ohio September 1996
3rd Printing – Boardman, Ohio May 1997
4th Printing – Boardman, Ohio November 1997
5th Printing – Boardman, Ohio February 1998
6th Printing – Warren, Ohio September 1998
7th Printing – Warren, Ohio December 1998
8th Printing – Warren, Ohio May 1999
9th Printing – Lancaster, California July 1999
10th Printing – Los Angeles, California February 2000
11th Printing – Las Vegas, Nevada June 2000
12th Printing – Las Vegas, Nevada November 2000
13th Printing – Las Vegas, Nevada April 2001
14th Printing – North Hollywood, California August 2001
15th Printing – Toronto, Ontario, Canada October 2001
16th Printing – Area 51, June 2002
17th Printing – Cap St Ignace, Quebec, Canada, February 2003
18th Printing – Cap St Ignace, Quebec, Canada, November 2003

TABLE OF CONTENTS PART ONE

TABLE OF CONTENTS PART TWO

IN THE BEGINNING..

"In many aspects, medical science in the United States is superior to every other country in the World. Yet, in terms of overall health care, freedom of choice, sophistication of many doctors, and education of the average American concerning Health, Exercise and Disease, we are lagging far behind many countries. Worse still, most of you don't even realize it." - *Thomas Edison*

It took me a long time to finally realize what people like Edison had been talking about. Harvey Kellogg, D.D. Palmer, Bernard Jensen, and others I emulated said one thing, and Arthur Jones, Joe Weider, Fred Hatfield others I also emulated said another. After researching a little more, they actually said a lot more of the 'same' things than I realized.

Discovering this required attention to detail. So at this very moment, I want you to commit to a specific time and place free of distraction that will allow you to study this manual in equal parts daily until you've read through it all. Treat this as the same sort of commitment you would make towards getting a better grade at school. Look at it as though you are studying for an advanced degree or higher level of knowledge. That is exactly what it is.

And you are expected to start the diet today, take notes, and use what you learn as soon as you have read it. Little by little, the results will come as you make one change after another and you won't feel like everything has changed all at once on you. Once you have read the book, read it again. Take a couple weeks each to read it the first few times, then read it again once a month until you're sure you've embedded it into your psyche. Then, once a year, go back and do it again or head to the website and discover what updates we now offer. Read your own notes. Compile an idea of what works for you so that it becomes second nature.

It'll be no time at all that your bad habits are gone and the good habits have you feeling and looking like you've always dreamed. I want your devoted attention and participation. I want you to get PSYCHED! I want you to read this OUT LOUD to yourself so you retain more of the material as we proceed. You will never again be bothered with volumes of literature, irrelevant data, fads and myths to get your answers! I say to you there is no need for science fiction when it comes to results either!

Just open your mind. Take a deep breath in. Exhale it. Regulate your thoughts. Set your sights and mind on your goals. Feel them. Become them. Dedicate yourself to them. Calculate your every action from here on out. Everything you do should be based solely on heading towards success. Visualize, taste and savor that. Feel it. Success is attainable! Welcome it, give color, texture and dimension. Allow it to happen by having so much vigor that you evoke a response so strong that it practically comes to life without you! Become thankful for your every waking moment because LIFE is a gift! Reach for the limits. No longer allow yourself to be set back. Forget your mistakes. Let them go. You have wanted to do this for a long time. It's YOUR time.

This program is for the young and old alike. It does not matter what your age is. Food goes in one end and out the other but what happens at all stops in between is what makes us today and tomorrow. Being fat or skinny only comes from your choice of eating habits. So does your health. If you do not want to eat as often or as much as I recommend, at least separate your foods accordingly and you will see results.

If you want to eat processed foods, things considered as junk by most definition, instead of taking in clean, nourishing and otherwise healthy foods, of course you will not look or feel the way you desire. Stress makes you fat even if you eat right. So relax and sleep more.

Worry and lack of sleep depletes us of certain nutrients that food cannot replace. Accepting that all things in life have both reason and solution. Know nothing needs done immediately, because most things rarely can be. Do this and you will make more progress than you have ever made in the past by living one quiet step at a time. Vegetarians especially need to learn food separation. That is the foundation of this program. By learning what is a carb, a fat and a protein, you can finally succeed as a vegetarian. Just because you only eat plants does not mean that you won't benefit by either having eggs and cottage cheese or eating your high protein, low carb foods separate from your high carb starches.

If you eat on the run and buy a lot of fast food, do what I do in a pinch, stop at the grocery store simply to enjoy tofu by itself. Are you a Barry Sears fans? Is 40-30-30 Nutrition your game? You like Bill Phillips and his Body For Life routine? Well, low fat, low carb, high protein, and even Zone dieters all must learn the food separation rules. If you want to follow a low fat plan, go right ahead. It's OK. Just make sure you take your Lemmon's Oil once a day. You need the essential fatty acids.

Those of you on Atkins, Protein Power or any other low carb program can still follow those routines only as long as you are willing to modify what you're doing a bit. Low carb diets aren't bad. But how they suggest you do it is bad. Trust me, exceeding 30 carbs a day hasn't made anybody I know fat. Once you begin to follow my suggestions, you will be surprised at the end of the day to see you are in fact, either in the correct Zone for your body weight after all or that your new low carb plan ala the KNOW HOW feels much better than anything you have attempted in the past. You do not need to be a fitness star, model, bodybuilder nor athlete to lose fat and look good. I hear it all the time...

"I don't want to be a muscle bound hunk or a breast implanted hottie, I just want to feel good and lose some fat." Not many people do want to be or do those things to look better and that's the idea. Odds are your goal is like mine. You want to be somewhere between where you are now and where the hunks and hotties are. I personally do not care what other people look like in their underwear; I only concern myself with how I feel each morning. I like the idea that I have total control over my own health and the fact that I can go to the beach anytime and feel confident about it. If you do happen to be someone who wants 'ripped' or 'shredded' then keep reading. I haven't forgotten about you!

Even children should learn food separation too so that they can avoid bad health and self esteem issues. I know kids are 'kids' or that 'teens' like to eat anything they choose... That doesn't make it right for you to let them. If your kid has acne, it isn't natural; it's due to their eating habits. And don't expect any visible progress for a while or overnight results if you weigh 400 pounds. You won't see abs for a couple hundred pounds. Sorry. Be patient. Junk foods contain artificial sweeteners and manufactured fats that alter the body's chemistry. It takes time for them to be eliminated from the system in order for results to show.

No matter the diet you want to follow, this book will make that diet work better for you. If you want to eat less carbs, then have less carbs in your diet. If you want more, then you can do that too. If you want to eat a little more low fat or even high fat, all I ask is that you follow the rules of food separation and you will still see results. However, the best results will always come by following this plan to the letter. It is up to the individual how they proceed, I merely lay the framework, but food separation applies to all diet plans.

Is this going to be as inexpensive as junk food sometimes is? Well, we all eat. Some afford more expensive foods and others cannot. But we all eat at some point during the day and even on a shoestring budget, you can get quite far on separating the baloney from the bread and replacing sodas with something cleaner from now on. By adhering to food separation, we eliminate digestive disorder so anyone can become healthy, fit and attractive. Bloating, pimples, headaches... It is all due to indigestion and it also goes away when you get on this program. Eliminating sugar, artificial sweeteners and lard is important on any 'diet' and doing so does not make food separation a fad nor only something for 'health' nuts. Does drinking more water than soda, juice or sweetened ice tea really sound unhealthy or like a fad? Just make the change and you will see the change.

Don Lemmon's KNOW HOW is no fad and just because you'll use this book as a guide for all your future eating habits doesn't mean you are on a diet either. Fads come and go. Diets do not work. I, and my 'food separation' program are not a fad nor going anywhere. We are here to stay. The foundation of the system, the 12 Food Groups, which you are about to learn about, will work for everyone because this is a lifestyle modification. The concept is leaps and bounds ahead of anything else you've used. It's something you can do and no one will know you're following... You're eating healthy foods because you're still having dark meat chicken, steak, pasta, cereal, etc.

Isn't it ironic though that natural foods are labeled as 'healthy' or only for health food 'nuts' because you chose not to eat donuts and pies? And to think you're made fun of for wanting to eat good food! Yeah, they laugh at you as if eating pastries and not being able to touch your toes without gasping for air makes someone 'cool'. WOW. And who said protein powders, meal replacement shakes or 'bars' are better for you than real food? Read the ingredients on those products. 'Frightening' doesn't begin to describe what they really do for you. Despite what they tell you in defense of their products, artificial sweeteners are poisons and anything you do that contradicts what we discuss will age you beyond your years.

How important is it for you to grow older gracefully? Have you seen someone at age 26 looking 40 already? 40 is not old but if you look 40 at 26 like many models I know do, you can be certain, when you turn 60 they're not going to look '40' unless they take better care of themselves. You do that already? Oh really? Why do you look or feel so much older than you really are? Stress? Oh please! Noah was stressed and he lived to be over 900. The body can handle stress... It was meant to. It's the repetitive undue stress that you do nothing to prepare for or repair that holds you back.

IF you ALLOW it to recover from stress, IF you really take care of yourself, THEN you will NOT age so quickly... If the outside is showing that you aren't aging gracefully, neither is the inside. Do not kid yourself, we ALL grow old. Nothing on God's green Earth is more important than human health. And let's be honest, as a society we are living longer, but we're doing it in nursing homes incapable of wiping our own butts. Improvements in medicine and education may keep us alive, but at what quality? Continue living the average lifestyle and you're inviting high blood pressure, heart disease, diabetes, osteoporosis, and cancer into your life. Get up. Eat right. Get active. Going to bingo isn't active. Weight lifting is active!

Oddly enough, Americans are the best fed people on Earth and yet we are also just about the laziest and most under-nourished Nation in the World too. So come on. Studies show that after we turn 30, the body naturally loses almost a pound of muscle a year and replaces it with over a pound of fat. They say the metabolism diminishes one percent a year. Imagine working off only half your optimal metabolism. If a 120 pound woman over 40 gains just five pounds of lean muscle, drops five pounds of fat, she inadvertently increases her caloric requirements by as much as 20%. This is a good thing. The faster the metabolism, the more fat your body fights to burn as opposed to store...

All she has to do to maintain this is exercise and eat right. You can't exactly resort back to your old bad habits and expect your body to stay fit you know. And the amount of muscle mass we carry is also a good indicator of our immune system, the strength of our bones, and the ability to withstand stress so we had better adapt a lifelong attitude towards maintaining ourselves before it's too late. Every little bit helps. Think of the animals you've seen in a zoo. Compare them to those that run free in the wild like the ones you see on TV. Zoo animals eat processed foods.

What you see them fed during the day is just for show and even if it is meat, it's not fresh meat, you can be certain of that. And since these animals do not have the room to run or a reason to (no food to catch), they do little work and exercise. They lose their muscle, strength, endurance, and LIFE SPANS.

It's amazing enough the direct correlation between man and wild animal. We too used to hunt our own foods but now we buy them from a store or have hot meals delivered to us prepackaged. We no longer run for our lives, look for shelter, chase our prey, and often we do not even exercise to make up for it. Nowadays we look for every way we can to relax, do nothing all day long, and make excuses all the while for the way we look and feel. Like caged animals, we have pouches under our bellies that hang. We couldn't fight to save our lives and get scared whenever someone says BOO. We are so sickly as a society that we worry we may have every single ailment that's advertised on late night TV. Isn't that pathetic? Yes, and this means if we are serious about our bodies, we must make a few changes. This goes for YOU too, Ms Fitness and Mr. America.

You are just as much at risk as anyone else. Especially you drug users. I spoke to a girl at the Ms. Olympia this year getting ready to compete that very night about her irregular heartbeat. It was too late that day for her to get off drugs, but it wasn't too late for her to begin becoming drug free the next day. I spoke with a bodybuilder at the Mr. USA also this year that had just urinated blood in the restroom during his steroid testing. Listen, if you have these problems now, it only gets worse. You really do not need to continue with this lifestyle. Do you find yourself visiting the doctor more often than ever before? It's not 'just' because of aging. It's because of the habits you have acquired until this day have FORCED YOU TO AGE.

IN CONSIDERATION OF THIS PROGRAM..

If you are on a 40-30-30 Nutrition plan or the Zone Diet… You WILL NATURALLY BE in the CORRECT 'zone' for your weight at the end of each day by separating your foods accordingly. If you follow the Atkin's diet or any other low carb ketogenic plan, just make sure all of your meals are protein, fat, and fibrous green vegetable based using the 3 to 1 protein to fat ratio rule. If you follow a 'low fat' or 'high carb' plan, make sure you keep all carb meals virtually non-fat and maintain protein meals at no more than 25% fat. This will keep things in a low fat perspective overall. Vegans, please maintain low carb protein and fat sources together, separate from high carb foods. While beans are not a protein, cottage cheese, eggs and tofu are. Oils and nuts do not go on or with starches....

If you are a teenager, you too must eat accordingly whether you are fat or not. Just because your friends eat a certain way doesn't mean it won't affect you later down the road. Know how you laugh at people who gain the Freshman 15 or the school alumni who are fat with thin hair at 30? That'll be you too because eating bad is what got them there.

What gives you gas does so because it doesn't digest properly, like burgers, fries and chips, will also not nourish you. Without nourishment, we do not grow, mature, nor age properly. For the elderly, those prescription medications you take will work better once you 'food separate' and your doctors will probably prescribe you less as we move forward. The body works best when all of its fuels are supplied and your motors are kept clean. Become efficient and you ARE efficient. Everyone is expected to exercise at least a couple times a week no matter which category they fall into. I only ask you to pick 3 exercises you know how to perform and set a schedule to do them. Don't be lazy.

Get up. Do something for yourself. Whether you are weak or strong, fast or slow, it doesn't matter. Your strength and speed is individual, just do what you can. In time, it all adds up to progress. Finally, if you 'food combine' that's great, but this isn't food combining. It's something better. This program explains why Fit For Life and Suzanne Somers have so many limitations. You see, this is the book I wish I could have had when I first took interest in nutrition and exercise.

Being misinformed and mislead obviously gets a person nowhere. It all began, in my youth, because I was frustrated and without proper guidance. I think of all the frustration that could be avoided. if a sound system was instilled in schools around the World today. But people are in their infancy of understanding how nutrition works and dieting isn't considered important I suppose. Well folks, consider yourselves briefed. It's now time for you to get what I call my 'Know How'… After I help you, maybe you can help me, get the word spread. 'Diet' is not a dirty word. Oh! When I say 'carbs' it is the same thing as carbohydrates… Its just slang! If you have any questions, email me via www.donlemmon.com My work thrives on your enquiries.

Without you telling me what is on your mind, I cannot make it more clear for you nor for others that come after you. Whatever your reason for being here is, you're here. So please take the time today and send me a question if you have one. But do me a favor and wait until you finish the book first. Do not be afraid to email me, just simply wait to do it once you have read everything. I understand some people will have some sincere questions because they truly do not understand, but too many people email me with questions that are already in the book prior to getting to those parts. Write your questions down as they arise, list the page your question stems from.

WHAT MY CLIENTS HAVE TO SAY..

You may think my clients were all Los Angeles, California bodybuilders or models because of the folk you have seen endorsing or representing my videos, my web site or this book, but they weren't. Nearly a third of them yes, were from California, but another third were from Ohio and the final third came from Las Vegas, NV (not to mention all the people I have worked with on the internet).

These are the three major geographical areas where I have spent the majority of my life. Every one of them wanted the same things. To look better. To feel better. To do it easily. To never revert back to their old selves. Their age groups? From teenagers to centurions. High school students and senior citizens. Who did I like working with the most? Definitely I especially enjoyed the seniors. Life is so funny. We start off curious. We get to a point where we think we know it all. We progress past that to actually believing we really do know it all. Then we begin to worry about what we do not know and somewhere in the later years, we finally come to relax about knowing some things that just do not matter.

I will never say to myself 'if I knew then, what I know now' because that's not as important as making the proper decisions with what we have to base them on and then doing something to follow through with it all. The testimonials I receive regarding the success of my program are by far one of the more popular sections of my website. I can see why. Sometimes I look at them myself and forget people are writing about ME. Check it out sometime. It will be motivating to discover people you emulate are using the KNOW HOW.

Actually, some of the people posted on my site were so appreciative of what the program did for them that they let me record phone interviews so we could make copies available to the public and we used to send them out for free in our supplement club packages. Everyone you meet in life will have radically different views stemming from their own personal experiences and backgrounds despite seeming so similar on the surface. Drop by the site and see if we have made these tapes available again or not.

That's about all you will need to know in order to go into this system and have the program work for you too. The following pages contain statements made about the KNOW HOW system from people who substantiate the fact. You can not only learn from those who have triumphed from their decisions but also from other people's mistakes. Thomas Edison is famous for saying, "I didn't succeed at creating the light bulb. I failed 10,000 times at determining what it took to create the damned thing." Isn't a program only as successful as the people using it? I think so. Ok, look at who my friends are and see what people are saying.

I think you'll be surprised by who's using The KNOW HOW system (not to mention where some of them have gotten using it). Thought those other programs are endorsed by the best? Guess again! I really can't think of a single program that can boast what I can. Nonetheless, look who we have here today. Enjoy the testimonials. I certainly did.

Mark Mortimer, actor, New York, NY - "I do not trust anyone other than Don Lemmon with my exercise and nutrition recommendations. When I first got on his diet, I was able to improve my appearance on what is considered by most people to be a sorry excuse of a workout schedule and eating way too much food. I could not believe how much of a difference separating foods and exercising only twice a week has made!"

Kristi Davis, masseuse, Burbank, CA - "Finally! I feel comfortable about the way I look in clothes, when I go out, and in the mirror after getting out of the shower! And I feel tough too! Nothing like having strength! Girl Power!'

Charles Sproule, martial artist, Truro, NS - "I have put on nearly 15 pounds of muscle using this system, and my wife is entering a bodybuilding show drug free looking as good as the competitors on steroids. Amazing!"

Kathy Faix, accountant, Youngstown, OH - "I've lost so many inches I'm almost embarrassed to discuss it! I've dropped a tremendous amount of fat and toned up REAL nice... Ask my husband Bob!" (She's lost 60 pounds of fat, gained 20 pounds of muscle in 6 months!)

Larry Wolf, contractor, Hubbard, OH - "I was over 300 pounds and literally carrying 100 pounds of excess fat when I met Don. When he told me I could eat what ever I wanted, I said 'Great!' Since he taught me how to basically separate some foods from others and while doing just that, now eating whatever I want, no catches, I've lost 80 pounds of fat. The strange this is, I am eating more than ever!"

Michelle Ralabate, fitness model, Miami, FL - "This is a program worth endorsing! I think it is great that Don is telling it like it is for a change! When he asked me then to be one of his primary spokeswomen for 1996 I immediately said HECK YEAH! This guy has done a lot to help those in this industry who wanted to reach their goals without drugs."

Tony Fabrizzio, real estate agent, Las Vegas, NV - "Don's program works. I entered a natural (drug free) bodybuilding contest in 1995 promoted by Denny Kakos and even though the judges said I was listed on score cards as the winner, I was asked to withdraw at the last minute. The competitors protested saying nobody could look as ripped (lean) as I did without taking drugs! Well, I tested drug free and I was drug free."

Dr. Jean Williams, professor, Youngstown, OH - "I'm 65 and since meeting Mr. Lemmon I have been eating three times the food I normally would, lost over thirty pounds of fat and my doctor has taken me off medication that I've been on for over 30 years as a diabetic with lupus. Don is tough, but I have made more progress in the 3 months separating foods than I have with all other trainers and programs combined! Plus, my stomach pains are gone. That alone was worth the effort!"

Dr. Gary Eversole, chiropractor, Las Vegas, NV - "I gained almost 30 pounds on the scale and dropped nearly a half a foot off my waistline. I eat what I want and only work out three times a week. Sometimes less on this system."

Laurie Donnelly, Ms Fitness America, Boulder, CO - "Don Lemmon certainly knows what he is doing! I was on a program similar to, but then again, nothing like Don's for my first year on television, which worked wonders. I and my two workout partners are giving Don a try without a bit of hesitation."

Kiko Ellsworth, actor, Studio City, CA - "I got The KNOW HOW and after a couple weeks I am toppling my previous strength records and can already see my abs. It works well enough I just shot my own calendar."

Grace Grimes, fitness model, Cincinnati, OH - "I was brought up on hours of training sessions like everyone else. Don really knows his stuff though. I am living proof that proper nutrition and consistent exercise are the keys to success, weight loss, and even maintaining yourself! This program works for post pregnancy too by the way!"

Kevin Pugh, chef, Detroit, MI - "I personally didn't think it were possible, but this is an eating plan that not only works but fits into an everyday lifestyle. I have personally lost over 80 pounds in just four months. I've known Don for ten years and I waited much too long to do this."

Heather Pariso, Ms Internet World, Dover, OH - "I not only do not worry about fat sneaking up on me, but if it did this is the obvious logical approach to losing it! It is nice to know I can now get away with exercising so little and yet eating so much."

Dr. Dave Williams, chiropractor, Las Vegas, NV - "I have never read a book that surprised me like this one. I feel Don has put together something the entire World needs to see. He has worked with my Bishop, a surgeon friend, my lawyer and all our families. I recommend Don Lemmon and his theories to anyone and everyone. Our 6:30 a.m. workouts are good times I will never forget."

Marjean Holden, Beastmaster actress, New Zealand - " Like you said, by manipulating the diet I didn't seem to notice a difference in my lifestyle. However, since doing as you suggested I'm really amazed at what my scale has told me! After losing several inches of blubber, I weigh the same as I did when I started but I look totally different! That must be muscle I gained while dropping fat right? Not bad."

Morris Sullivan, film producer, Toluca Lake, CA - "I was insulted at how simple the plan is. My strength at age 76 has never been better. I have gained 10 pounds of muscle though it looks like more and I am not even trying to lose fat but I am. Not bad for an old man. And my blood tests show me to be a much younger man!"

Kelly Boling, secretary, Washington, DC - "I feel absolutely terrific. But even better than that, my mental acuity has improved tremendously. I swear I woke up this morning a dress size smaller too. My pants are fitting loosely, my stomach's flatter, my arms and legs look leaner, all in a month."

Dr. Robert Zeravica, chiropractor, Los Angeles, CA - "I honestly agree with every thing in this book. With so many nutritional programs on the market, I am amazed at how Don compiled all of this. Don's work should be required reading for all health care providers."

Nadia Alterio, BA Psychology, Las Vegas, NV - "In the first 2 weeks I followed the program I made changes in my diet and health that I didn't realize were possible. For the longest time I believed I was lactose intolerant but now I know that I am not. The layers of body fat I have shed without using 'fat burners' is amazing!"

Artie Kaikou, martial artist, Akron, OH - "My strength is becoming incredible! Thank you. At first I didn't think it made sense but now it makes so much sense. I would have never achieved what I have without this KNOW HOW system. I tried for 10 years to get where I was able to get in just 10 weeks. I was 40 pounds lighter 3 months ago and I honestly feel I am not done yet. I can achieve anything now!"

Grace DeLaRosa, newscaster, Oahu, HI - "There is nothing like knowing that you look good and have your health all year long. Too many times in the past I didn't want to do a shoot because I wasn't feeling my best. I guess you could say being on the Know How is like having extra money in your pocket!"

Brian Blazek, bartender, Henderson, NV - "I have added over 50 pounds to my bench, squat and dead lifts, 60 to my rows and gone from 45 to 65 pounds on my curls. Is this really possible? To top it all off, I seem to be literally repelling body fat as I get leaner and leaner by the moment! As if it couldn't get better, my first cover offer came today!"

Suzanne Clark, TJ Clark Co, St George, UT - "I got The Don Lemmon program and right away, I couldn't believe how good the book turned out to be. I read it, followed it, asked a few questions and then was on my own without fear of failing. It was almost too easy. "

THE TEN STEPS TO RECOVERY QUICK START..

1) Before bed, place a glass of water by your nightstand. Take a sip whenever you wake up in the middle of the night and finish the glass as soon as you wake up in the morning. Always drink water upon awakening, then again between and after (but not before) meals, and even before bed.

2) When the alarm RINGS it is time to get up -NOT hit the snooze button for more rest! IMMEDIATELY after having your water begin eating! Food is your top priority. It doesn't matter if your day starts at 2 o'clock in the afternoon. Get up and eat. If you think you have no time, move your tail a little faster. Make time. Eat before you do anything else including going poo-poo.

3) Be sure to eat again at least every three hours following this meal. Try not to let more than 2 1/2 hours go between ending and starting your feedings. Skipping a meal is ALWAYS worse than over eating. It slows your metabolism. Eat often just like a baby does and NEVER skip a feeding.

4) Alternate your meals between four protein and vegetable meals and two carbohydrate based low fat meals each day. If you are afraid to eat fat or carbs, at least separate the animal protein foods you have from all starches into different sittings. For now, all meals should be equal in calories. Never have two carbohydrate-based meals in a row.

5) Schedule meals so you finish eating 1 1/2 hour before and again 1/2 hour after exercise. Have proteins before training and carbohydrates after. This is the opposite of what you heard in the past but it works. REPEAT: Carbs are for AFTER and proteins are for BEFORE your workout sessions. Only drink water during exercise. There are no exceptions. Protein before, carbs after. Nothing else will work.

6) Exercise with weights possibly Monday, Wednesday, and Friday this week then only Monday and Thursday next week. Determine what's best for you, but these days are typical. You can select any 5 non-consecutive days every 2 weeks to workout that you like. You can do 3 sessions a week or 2 sessions. 2 are all you need and 3 isn't always better. Perform one exercise per muscle group for up to 10 total sets a session or try the 3 sets of 3 exercises routine. End each session with 12 minutes of cardio.

7) Write down everything you do. When you weight lift, log the weight you use and how many repetitions you performed. If you can lift something more than 10 reps, you need to use more weight the next time and if you can't, keep using it until 10 are possible. When you use aerobic machines, log the distance you go. Do not try for more and more time. Try for further distances in the same amount time. Huff and puff!

8) Get 8 hours of sleep. If possible, beginning prior to 11 p.m. No matter what, lay down for 8 hours a day even if it's in segments. No matter who you are, you know as well as I do that 8 hours on your back is easy enough to perform even in spurts through out the day. I pulled it off with 2 jobs, full time study and commuting.

9) Keep your body in mental, physical, emotional and spiritual alignment. Say a thankful prayer daily. If you promise not to lie, steal, swear, lust or get angry with people, then you will avoid 90% of what causes a person stress any given day.

10) Look challenge in the eye. I do. And I always walk away proud... Take this book with you to work or along on travel. When you come up with ideas, make notes and tell me about them online later. I want you to become so involved in this program it reverses, de-programs and alters every thing that you think you know. I want you to realize it is because everything you thought you knew about fitness in the past has been wrong.

THE 12 FOOD GROUPS: PROTEIN MEALS

I think it is easier to learn a little about 12 things than it is to learn a lot about 4. The four food groups aren't put together right anyhow and I think it is time we have it simplified. I know 12 sounds confusing at first, but the foods conveniently all fall into only 12 different categories. And this is what makes it so easy. In nature, all protein sources of substantial content are virtually carb free. They are also sources of fats.

Eggs have a white (protein part) and a yolk (fat part), meat has muscle (protein part) and marble (fat part), etc. Carbohydrate foods tend to be low protein and devoid of fat unless the company processing them added oil or lard to the mix. This is important to understand because the body only knows how to process foods as they come in nature. By simply allowing the body the ability to recognize whether what you eat is a protein and fat, or the opposite, a low protein, nonfat carbohydrate food, miracles occur. Confused? Don't be. That's why I created the 12 Food Groups. Now all food selection is made easy. Let's begin…

You are about to discover the truth about foods and their benefits here, but you will also learn simple calorie tips so all you need to know is the approximate measures of your selections to succeed. If you are wondering how I get these caloric figures, I read labels. I discovered over time that most foods in their 'like' groups contain the same calories pound for pound, but I still suggest you read labels for a while to get to know your own selections. All foods contain proteins, carbohydrates and fats.

When you read a label, remember carbohydrates and proteins both have 4 calories a gram and fat has nine. That doesn't mean carbs and proteins are equal in energy production or that fat is evil. However, while a gram of carb has 4 calories, it only burns

4 calories while digesting. Carbohydrates almost 'melt' as opposed to burn and this is why they digest so quickly. Fat too burns it's weight in calories. However, protein, being of first importance, contains 4 calories a gram but burns almost 6 calories a gram once eaten! So protein SPEEDS your metabolism JUST by eating it! But not if you eat it with carbs! That goes against nature! Still, carbs are important too! They are simply of no use if you eat them with fats and... Protein. You need them. Proteins contain and create enzymes, rebuild tissues and the porphyrin molecules that assist hemoglobin in carrying oxygen around.

Low protein diets lead to weak hearts. Prothrombin, thrombin, fibrin and fibrinogen from proteins heal wounds and clots blood. Eat protein, prevent strokes. Lipids from proteins line our mitochondrias that create electrical energy (some say our very souls) from within. You'll think more clearly. And lipoproteins transport bad fats out of the body. You need protein to reduce cholesterol. I do not agree with the methods used to kill animals these days nor how they are raised. But this is why I am careful with the brands I use and purchase.

I am not going to say you 'must' eat meat, but I will say you must get sufficient protein. Eggs and cottage cheese is a staple in my diet although I do not eat as much meat as I did in the past... Before we continue, there is something I want to add. I am often asked whether the foods in the 12 Food Groups are either alkaline or acidic. It may seem like that is important and it is not that it isn't, but it is not nearly as significant as the other nutritional info we'll cover. Still, since you're dying to know what I am talking about, the terms alkaline and acid 'ashes' refer to what's remaining after processing a particular food.

When you take food and have it dried in a lab to a point it becomes an ash, the characteristics of that ash is either acid, alkaline or neutral. Potatoes, legumes and vegetables are pretty much all alkaline foods. Grains and animal products are acidic. Fats are neutral. Some alkaline foods like legumes, melons, broccoli and tubers (potatoes) reduce the acidity of your gut and urine. Foods like sour fruits increase it. What you eat determines if you are off or on and hot or cold. You need a balance of all things in your life.

Acid foods are the body's accelerators and alkaline foods put on the brakes. If the brakes work, but the accelerator doesn't, the car won't move. If the pedal is to the floor and nothing is there to slow you down, you're headed for trouble. Understand? This is a sticky subject if you want to know the truth. For instance, some people with more acidity in their GI tracts must be given hydrochloric acid as a remedy. Others will require an alkaline bile salt instead (pruitus ani). Since the effects of these two substances are exactly the opposite of one another, it is easy to see where the necessity for a medical diagnosis fits in.

At this point, whether this program seemingly meets your standard and fits into your schedule or not is relevant. If you are going to eat at all (once, twice, three or even ten times a day), you can still make the appropriate decisions to eat right based upon these 12 Food Groups. You will learn all that matters in making sure you have balance in the 12 Food Groups. I have made things very easy to implement if you will just follow my lead. Saying that learning some new tricks are too hard, too much, or a burden and inconvenience in any way is a joke. You eat anyhow so from now on, just follow my lead and eat right when you do. That's not too much to ask. At least then you will see and feel the difference before making the blind decisions of the past that got you here to begin with.

FOOD GROUP #1 – EGGS

Attention Vegans: Eggs are not baby chickens. A rooster must fertilize the hen to make babies. This is why egg farms do not have roosters around. And since eggs are not from cows, we do not consider them part of the dairy group. Eggs supposedly contain 'the most complete source of protein available' but they are a still a little hard to digest and because of this, eggs should be not only cooked but eaten before anything else in your meal. The only raw eggs I eat come directly from a farm. A larger whole egg (white and yolk together) contains about 6 grams of protein, 4 grams of fat and 60 calories.

The white alone has 5 grams of protein and 20 calories. The yolk contains, 1 protein gram and 4 in fat. Despite the high quality nutrients, which are essential amino acids (in the protein), lecithin and cholesterol, I recommend having only one yolk for every three or four whites that you eat. I love farm fresh egg yolks though. Because farm fresh eggs haven't been pasteurized, they have their enzymes intact so you can eat more of them. So unless you get your eggs from a farm, get all your other fat calories from Food Groups 6 and 7. If you didn't know it until now, cholesterol free diets don't work.

You need fats like that in egg yolks. Only by EATING cholesterol regularly is the body able to control it's HDL and LDL levels. Ironically, egg yolks not only contain cholesterol themselves, but they also contain the highest natural source of cholesterol mobilizers. The supplement industry has made GAZILLIONS off these "fat burning" compounds found in eggs (although they now choose to use less effective and less expensive soy forms). The compounds are lecithin, choline and inositol and all three are found in virtually every fat burning supplement made in the past 20 years.

Here I sit telling people to eat eggs for a more natural source of these nutrients and you're refusing to eat the best tasting part? The yolks. What, are you nuts? This means DEVILED EGGS ARE NOW ACCEPTABLE! Here's a boiling tip for you to make them. Poke a pinhole in the round end. Put a TB of salt, a

TB of vinegar and a cup of chicken broth in the water. Use a cooking thermometer to boil your eggs for 25 minutes at 180 degrees. DING! Done!

What does an egg meal look like for me? I usually mix about a TB (tablespoon) of whole raw cream in every 8 egg whites and 2 1/2 yolks, which makes them fluffy when they're cooked. I stir it up with sea salt and black pepper then place them covered in the fridge overnight. The next morning I scramble my eggs without needing to waste the time to crack and separate shells. Sometimes I use low fat cheese. Depending on what else you like, I also dice mushrooms, green peppers, and onions twice a week that I keep in Tupperware to put in these eggs too. I may have some tea on the side, but I do not have bread, cereal, milk or juice with my eggs.

TIPS: There is no secret to knowing which eggs contain salmonella. Make sure each dozen you buy have no cracked shells first. After that, refrigerating your eggs will prevent bad bacteria from multiplying. The only way to kill salmonella microbes is to heat them. That means no raw eggs unless they are truly farm fresh. This is especially important for people with weaker immune systems like the elderly, those with disease, pregnant women, and pets. Experts also say that "free-range" chicken eggs may be even more likely to harbor bacteria. When chickens are allowed to run around the barnyard together, they eat each other's poop and that breeds a bad egg. If you crack open an egg with blood in it, throw it away. Do not eat it.

FOOD GROUP #2 – SEAFOOD

Seafoods I like are sea bass, haddock, pollock, sashimi tuna, flounder, perch, swordfish, halibut, orange roughy, albacore tuna, salmon, lake trout and yellow fin. They are all good protein sources. Try to avoid the higher sodium ocean water types if you have hypertension. Check with your 'fish'ician if you have questions. Some fish are high in toxins. Usually the fatty ones caught near polluted waters and the like. Most seafood is typically low in fat (averaging 23 grams of protein and just 3 grams of fat per quarter -1/4- pound). The rule with low fat proteins is that they require a little added fat to digest most efficiently. Any oil from Food Groups 6 or 7 would work, but add them only AFTER cooking, not before.

Cooking destroys the good things in fat and that's what makes them poisonous to your digestive tract. Dead fats build toxins in the intestines, stress your immune system and lead to weakened lungs and allergies. Good fats do the opposite. It is crucial that you at least adhere to this ONE law of fats. Do not ever over heat them.

If you can't stand to eat fats at room temperature, or barely heated, either learn to do so or do not eat them at all. If you have been eating what you thought was good fat up until now, this is one reason why it hasn't helped yet. Sorry, fried foods are terrible for you and not just because they are breaded. Never eat anything fried and breaded. Grains, flours, fruits, potatoes, rices, and sodas have no place in a proper seafood meal. Even when we get sushi we only have fish and seaweed with soy sauce, ginger and wasabi. No rice. When we hit the sushi buffets we load up on spicy tuna hand rolls (no rice) sometimes exclusively!

FOOD GROUP #3 – LAND ANIMALS

Animal meat is good for you, and many of the flesh foods (like seafood) are low in fat which also means you will be required to add oils to them as well for better digestion. I know, I hear all the vegetarians screaming, "Dead animals?" I say "Dead plants?" The life may be gone from animal meat, but just like a plant, the nutrients remain as long as the food is fresh and wasn't left to spoil. So just as a piece of meat spoils, a vegetable spoils too. It's the same process. Sure there are too many drugs and the killing methods used on animals these days are sometimes less than honorable, but there are WAY more pesticides and chemicals in our plants than hormones in our meats. We need the nutrients found only in meats to live. Use your own discretion in making purchases, but at least once a week, gnaw away at something formerly attached to a bone.

Birds, poultry, red meat, 4 legged creatures and other common sources of animal flesh, trimmed of all visible fat and skin (there is no benefit to eating the excess marbles of fat or skin, that's where many of the toxins are stored), contain per quarter (1/4) pound, almost 25 grams of protein, less than 5 grams of fat and around 135 calories on the average.

Protein exclusively from meat is not essential to this or any program if you will at least eat eggs and cheese (although one meal a day of meat never killed anyone). If you currently have ulcers, supplement with pepsin (this will assist in protein digestion until your body heals itself) and drink comfrey tea (a special herbal tea, very inexpensive) with a small amount of raw cream each morning. This combo may also assist to heal a weakened stomach lining.

Our favorite? Fresh grilled steaks or chicken with sea salt, pepper, and grilled green beans or a Caesar salad devoid of croutons. No bread, no potatoes, no wine, no carbs. We save our carbs for a separate meal.

Essentially, it is best for you to eat your proteins first. Take your chicken for example, grill it up if you want, baste it or whatever. Do anything but put sugar or breading on it. Keep carbohydrates completely away from your proteins even while seasoning. That little bit of breading the waitress says won't hurt you, will. So just season it, cook it and eat it. Next, after it's down, get some green vegetables in your belly with a little cheese or oil on them. The reason we do this is because the body releases more enzymes to break down fat than it does to break down protein. That's how the body works in nature.

Some land animal meats are higher in fat than they are in protein, but to reverse the effects of fat storage that we have all suffered, we must reduce the fat in those selections. I.E. Remove the skin, any visible marbles of fat… You need to consume just enough fat, not a lot, to inhibit those excess fat enzymes from attacking the amino acids from the protein. I eat chicken thighs and legs trimmed and skinned more than I do breasts for this reason. That reduces the fat content quite a bit. After it's eaten, I have spinach or broccoli with butter on it. I might have a spring salad with spinach and Lemmon's Oil mixed with feta cheese. Whatever I have, it will be AFTER I have the protein.

As far as anti-biotics or any other pharmaceuticals used on cattle or chickens go, trust me when I say that YOU take more drugs than your meat did before reaching your plate. Organic meat is no different. All cattle companies use some sort of pesticide directly applied to the animals as a necessary step in ridding intestinal parasites such as blood worms and tape worms. It is illegal in the U.S. for drugs to be used in harmful doses.

FOOD GROUP #4 – ORGAN MEAT

Organ meats are another GREAT source of both protein AND fat if bought free of anti-biotics and steroids. Vegetarians, please don't stop here, you don't have to eat anything you do not want to. I have other food tips coming up that will help you through this without meats. Organs are things like tongues, hearts, tripe, brains, lungs, and whatever else from the insides of your favorite critter. Organ meats contain various nutritional co-factors that aid in our overall health that muscle tissue and vegetables do not provide.

Their calorie counts vary widely. You DEFINITELY need a calorie handbook to check out the particulars of the ones you choose. I personally use 'desiccated' (de-fatted and dehydrated) organ meats that are put into capsule form because they supply me with those nutritional co-factors other foods do not and this way I do not need to eat this stuff either.

I do not enjoy the taste of some organ foods. But prepared properly... They certainly can be tasty. I really like my liver and onions. No ice tea, no soda, no fries, no carbs are to be eaten with your organ meats. Man, a good liver with mixed peppers and onions just can't be beat. Liver is a food that is considered a blood builder and improves the appearance of your skin.

Over weight people who eat liver tend to look healthier than those who do not eat it for this reason... Did you also know, historically, organ cuts used to be the most valued parts of the kill? Meat was literally tossed aside to the dogs instead! Go figure!

FOOD GROUP #5 – DAIRY PRODUCTS

Dairy foods are sources of proteins, fats, and carbohydrates. After this discussion you will understand how an innocent mistake like drinking 2% milk with your cereal can turn into a major disaster. Some dairy foods are protein and fat sources, some are protein and carb sources. We are most familiar with milks, yogurts and cheeses and we will discuss milks and yogurts first. For digestive purposes, never drink milk or eat yogurts that have fat in them. They should be considered CARB foods, eaten only nonfat and separate from your meats and fats.

Always buy yogurts with no added sugar or artificial sweeteners added. Milk and yogurts are generally about 8 grams of protein and 12 to 16 carbohydrates per 8 ounces. This includes unflavored yogurts, acidophilus (a healthy, spoiled milk product that contains a lot of friendly bacteria that are good for the digestive tract), butter milk, custard, and any other dairy product high in carbs. Buy them as low fat as possible. If there is more than a gram of fat per serving, do not have it.

Follow these rules and you just might not be lactose intolerant after all. The natural sugars in milk simply cause digestive complications leading to the belief that you are lactose intolerant as a result of eating whole fat products (you're probably catching on, you can't mix fat and carbs when you eat). Even if carbs and fats are found naturally together in milk, this isn't a mistake of GOD. The complications are caused by a mistake of man. It's pasteurization. Scientists thought pasteurization was a good thing at first because it lowered the bacteria count of raw milk. However, 48 hours later with all the acidophilus, good bacteria and enzymes gone (this is what makes milk sour), the bad bacteria is left unchallenged so it returns and skyrockets to toxic levels!

Therefore, pasteurization may not be so cool after all. All the farting, belching, intestinal cramps, GAS, constipation and other problems are avoidable if you'll make the appropriate changes. Why do they do this? Because raw milk lasts about one week and pasteurized lasts at least two. The manufacturers of these foods say 'so what' if this process kills both the good AND the bad bacteria, just as long as it allows the foods to stay on a store shelf a little longer without spoiling. This is what prevents them from needing to buy food to replace what spoiled on them and ups the odds you're buying spoiled food anyhow.

Without all the good natural things foods before being chemically altered, we end up sick and internally distressed by using pasteurized dairy products. So, unless you use raw milk, don't drink whole milk. And if you have raw milk, drink some by itself. Whatever brand you use, sip it, don't chug it and take a good 20 minutes to finish a cold glass. Yogurt. To turn milk into a yogurt, you must first sterilize the milk then plant a 'culture' in it. The culture sours the milk, which forms the yogurt. Natural soured milk is much better for this reason as the acidophilus is still intact.

However, people with chronic pains and intestinal parasites are suggested to avoid all milk products and begin eating black walnuts or pomegranates, which break the parasites down. A good meal with dairy for me would be oatmeal, blueberries and nonfat milk or a bagel with a fruit spread and nonfat yogurt. If I want cheese instead.... Dairy products that are not high in carbohydrates but are good sources of protein and fat, while remaining devoid of almost all carbs, include sour cream, real butter (NEVER margarine), natural mayonnaises and my favorite, cheese. When I say cheese, I am talking hard cheeses that break easily and aren't creamy. I like provolone, smoked Gouda, feta on Greek Salads, cheddar, mozzarella, jack, Swiss, Parmesan, Romano and such. The easiest to digest cheeses are anything crumbly. I always have a little cheese with my meats and salads. The calcium in cheese balances the phosphorus levels in meat. A little cheese can and probably should be had with meat or eggs anytime you eat them.

Most contain around 7 grams of protein, 1 or 2 carbohydrates, 8 grams of fat, and about 110 calories an ounce. I try to get low fat sources. The only difference is less fat. In regards to butter and creams, they are fats so make sure you read the labels and know how much you're having when you select them. I put cheese in my eggs, on my salads, and sometimes on steamed veggies. I never put cheese on breads or potatoes... The only reason that you might think you are lactose intolerant is because you have problems with processed cheeses that are mixed with sugars to make them creamy. Rarely do whole cheeses cause digestive disorder. I would suggest only eating cheese that crumble or breaks for the time being such as goat, feta, and bleu etc if you are certain you're currently sensitive to dairy products. I bet your sensitivity goes away in no time.

Another of my favorites: Nonfat cottage cheese with Lemmon's Oil, ginger, allspice, nutmeg and cinnamon. No fruit, no berries, no brown sugar, no carbs or bagels… It's a high protein food. So no carbs allowed other than the 2 or 3 grams found naturally in it. I add just enough oil in it for a 3 to 1 ratio of protein to fat. A cup and a half of nonfat cottage cheese has 45 grams of protein so I add a TB of oil, which is 15 grams of fat to balance things out. 15 times 3 is 45. The same goes for whey protein. Whey protein is in fact a dairy protein too. Considering it is low fat naturally, it should be mixed with a third the amount of calories in fat grams from cream to digest properly. Yes, this is safe and will not raise your cholesterol levels.

I personally freeze my cream in ice cubes, 2 TB in each cube or so and then I add them to the whey when the time comes. In fact, there was a point in time I was using well over a quart of cream a day doing this with no ill effects.

But you see, the decision of what dairy product to eat is based upon what else you would plan to eat at that meal. For instance, cream cheese is bought fat free if you are using it on breads or bagels. This is because carb meals are meant to be fat free. But regular whole fat cream cheese goes great on meats or veggies as a dip. Sour cream can be bought fat free for potatoes but you'll use whole fat for meats and veggies. And sorry, but it goes without saying that unless you can find an ice cream or salad dressing that is both fat free and contains no artificial sugars (no added table sugar at all either), it's off limits. Too many low fat versions of snacks and dressings are just sugar filled nightmares waiting to fatten you up.

Note: When you are down to losing those last 5 or 10 pounds, I would suggest dropping all dairy products that are not pasteurized with the exception of a little real butter with fibrous veggies at meat meals. Contact a farm near you for cream and milk if your grocer hasn't been helpful. Not all health food store employees have a clue what you're talking about cause they don't walk the walk...

If you want what we consider to be the best blend of protein powder available, visit: www.completeproteinpowder.com

FOOD GROUP #6 – NUTS AND SEEDS

Nuts and seeds are regarded by vegetarians to be sources of protein and thought of by weight watchers as too fatty, but they also contain a considerable amount of carbs too, so low carb dieters shun many of these tasty treats. Who is right? Well, I call them fats because that is the predominant nutrient inside of them. There's two or three times more fat than protein but more protein than carbs, so... So, folks, they are FATS... But still, are they fattening? Only if you're eating creamy butter blended or roasted with hydrogenated oils, sugar or corn syrup as most name brands do. Plain nuts and seeds are good for you and hardly fattening. Phyto-nutrients, the powerful healing components found within plant foods that, like the ones in herbs, have regenerative properties. These factors are also found in some nuts and seeds, which stimulate you to burn fat.

Chestnuts, cashews, peanuts, almonds, pecans, macadamias, walnuts, pistachios, pine nuts, sunflower seeds, etc. are great choices. Go for the dry roasted only if you cannot purchase them in the raw. An ounce (1 oz.) of nuts/seeds or nut/seed butter contains on the average around 7 grams of protein, 7 carbs, 14 grams of fat and about 182 calories. DEFINITELY read your labels and look for coconut, cottonseed or any other oils used in the packaging.

Now, here's the deal. I take a half dozen different nuts and seeds then blend them in my peanut butter machine. When it is done, I mix in whey protein and Lemmon's Oil. From there, I have a higher protein, healthy fat spread, that I put on celery for a wonderful mid day snack. Just watch yourself. A little goes a long way. TIP: People with parasites should be sure to have black walnuts in their diet because that particular nut's enzymes inhibit parasite growth.

Remember, fats do not go with starches. This means no peanut butter sandwiches unless your grocer carries that virtually nonfat peanut spread I use! Soybeans fall into this category if you look at the caloric content of soy products. Tufo for instance has a 2 to 1 ratio of protein to fat. The carbs are pretty low. Some brands are bought fat free. I buy one carton that is fat free, then add it to some 'whole fat' brand I also like, stir fry them up with bok choy, peppers, mushrooms, etc, and love the feeling of eating clean, vegetarian food. Sometimes I have a handful of roasted soybeans (which are a little higher in fat) and wash them down with a glass of whey protein.

Soy isoflavones are a hot topic these days. These 'isoflavones' are really phytoestrogens, which in turn are simply plant chemicals that mimic the estrogen found normally in humans. Plant estrogens are thought to be beneficial in controlling estrogen fluctuations during and after menopause but they also compete for the same estrogen receptors as your natural hormones which block estrogen from doing it's job. This promotes estrogen based breast tumors.

So like it or not, too much soy can throw hormones out of balance, causing thyroid issues, irregular menstrual cycles and even infertility. A serving of tofu, miso, tempeh, soymilk or soybeans have about 40 mg of isoflavones each. Soy hot dogs or cheese have lower amounts of isoflavones because of processing. Soy sauce has almost none. Most clinical studies that show a problem with excess isoflavones had subjects ingesting 300 mg or more a day. Beneficial results without complication occur using 50 to 100 mg. I personally use soy as a food but I don't exceed 100 mg a day. But we all know someone who suffers one or more rather odd or troublesome health issues. The majority of these people are women and vegetarians… Go figure.

FOOD GROUP #7 – FATS AND OILS

Listen, let's get something straight, high fat diets do not work like they say they do and this program is NOT a high fat diet. However, without fats in the diet at all, oxygen can't reach your brain. So for those of you who are fat deficient, grab a tablespoon of Lemmon's Oil, put your thinking cap on, and let's learn a little something about that taboo nutrient you feel is so scary. For those of you who do eat fat, keep in mind, you may still be doing something wrong, keep reading.

For instance, you can't eat fats before eating protein. You should instead eat them during or after having the protein food. You also shouldn't exceed the recommended fat intake I've suggested either. If you do, the fats you eat may inhibit the secretion of the digestive juices upon the protein. This leaves them poorly broken down. And if the right amount of fat at your protein meal is not naturally contained in your protein food source, you must always add more afterwards along with some green vegetables like a salad, green beans, spinach or broccoli. The same applies to greens as the fats. They are best eaten after, not before the meal.

I realize these veggies have a little carbohydrate in them but it's a fibrous carbohydrate, not a starchy carbohydrate. Fibrous vegetables offer added benefit by delaying the potential adverse reaction of fat enzymes upon your proteins by binding with the fat. As long as you keep that 3 to 1 ratio of fat to protein I mentioned in mind when adding fat to a meal, you'll be fine. Yes, I am sure the little bit of fat in your canned tuna or chicken breast is not enough to assist digestion. Why? Since we take the skin off of our meats because that is where animals and fish store toxins, we obviously lose some fat content.

This is good, but the fat needs to be replaced. We're being smart about it and adding something healthy like real butter on the greens (salted or unsalted doesn't matter) to replace the unhealthy. Just do not cook with butter or any other oil with the exception of possibly using olive, sesame or coconut oil under medium heat at best. High heat destroys fats and turns them poisonous instead of nutritious. Technically it hydrogenates them. Cook your food first, then pour the oil or butter on AFTERWARDS. Butter? Yes. We will NEVER use margarine on this program.

One of THE BIGGEST misconceptions in the WORLD is that margarine somehow reduces cholesterol because it contains none. Butter contains natural cholesterol AND cholesterol metabolizing nutrients. Margarine does not. Margarine, like the coconut oil used in commercial baked goods, is made from hydrogenated oils, the body's silent enemy. The coconut oil I use for cooking is not the same oil as in baked goods and meal replacements. That stuff has been hydrogenated too. Ours is unprocessed… You want fats that are nourishing and build up your health, not deplete it.

What other fats do I use? I use my own oil blend, Lemmon's Oil, for the most part. 1 TB is perfect for most salads and meeting your essential needs. Treats? I use 3 TB of heavy whipping cream in my occasional Java. I look forward to my cup of 'Joe' because of that cream. By the way, I used to be a coffee-a-holic but I cut back once and my adrenal system became stressed. If you get tired after having coffee, it's time for a 'coffee' break. I feel fantastic having coffee only mid afternoons, 3 days a week, never in the mornings, nor late at night. If we do have morning coffee, it is one of those naturally caffeine free brands. De-caffienated coffees have bleaches in them.

If you are an addict, trust me, only once you wean off caffeine will you know how well the body actually works. Caffeine limits your body's ability to function properly. Until you clean yourself up, you really don't remember how energetic the body can be. Dressings! You can sparingly use fatty dressings on salads if they are eaten with proteins (eggs or meats) devoid of croutons and pasta or other carbs. By fatty, I mean a dressing that has only a couple carbohydrates in it and is mostly fat like bleu cheese, ranch, or even Caesar. If you decide to have a salad with a carbohydrate meal, use an unsweetened nonfat dressing instead. Read labels so you can stay within these parameters.

To keep from going over board, have the dressing on the side. Dip your fork in it before taking a bite of salad and you'll finally control unwitting overloading. A tablespoon serving of oil, butter or dressing generally contains almost 14 grams of fat, no carbs, no protein and 126 calories. The official Don Lemmon "Lemmon's" Oil, is a perfect blend of several different oils that contains 50% Omega 3, 20% of both Omega 6 and Omega 9 then 10% more from other essential fat sources. For more, see lemmonsoil.com. It has a thick feel, a nourishing dark look and a fresh nutty taste.

No other blend has any comparison whatsoever to this oil and what it does for you. A tablespoon or two of Lemmon's Oil essential fatty acids a day, will be just enough to keep the doctor at bay. This stuff is awesome. It regulates your hormones, your cells, everything. The special fats we use carry oxygen to our cells too. This makes them more receptive to your other nutrients. So you need them. The body wasn't designed to live off what it makes from other food sources. While it's true the body can make Omega 3 from the fat found in soybean oil this process skips a beat in the natural biochemistry of the body.

Just like we humans may have similar bits and pieces that cannot be exchanged, we can't equally exchange blood types any better than can we get the 'same' substances from exchanging DIFFERENT food groups. All things require or sometimes do not require a more or less of a complicated process for processing so you must remain aware of each food substance you consume. And I don't want anybody to think I mean medium chain triglycerides when I say ESSENTIAL Fatty Acid because the hype behind MCT's are unfounded. You may be curious about MCT or Medium Chain Triglyceride oils. I would rather you not use extra MCT's.

They are not essential fats. They are also unavailable as the effective 8-chain oils they used to be. They need to be taken in amounts too large to be financially feasible. Using them even just before a workout for energy doesn't assist you in burning extra body fat so why bother? MCT's are simply saturated fats derived from tropical oils.

Despite what you may hear, what you will find on the market these days is a single 10-chain lipid, which has no fat burning characteristics. In fact, they will only MAKE you fat, upset your stomach and deplete you of your essentials. You can't even buy MCT's in America that do what you expect of them without a prescription.

TIP: If you find at any time during the day you crave sugar, this is a signal of either you are not eating enough or that you are actually burning body fat. If you 'give in' and eat carbohydrates when you crave carbohydrates, you will shut off your fat burning mechanisms. If you start craving pizza, ice cream, pasta etc. now you know why. But you probably didn't know you can eat anything and the cravings will disappear. So be wise, have protein and fat instead from now on. If I crave sugar when I am done eating protein and fats, I know I didn't have enough fat at my meal. In fact, if I begin craving sugar at any time that tells me my blood sugar is low.

I know at that moment my body is going to begin BURNING fat but not if I eat sugar during a craving. If I do that, the fat burning shuts down. Listen to your body and you can't lose. When you are looking for essential fatty acids, I use not only my own Lemmon's Oil but also several other fat sources individually because I truly enjoy their taste. Almost daily, I have wheat germ oil, pumpkin seed butter, coconut butter, olive oil, chili oil, sesame oils and others. I only purchase them from one company, the same that creates mine. If you are interested in viewing my complete grocery list online, simply send me an email and I will direct you to it.

Keep something else in mind; the oil you buy does not need to be in glass bottles to protect it. The additional weight of glass increases the shipping rates, therefore cost of your oils. It isn't that plastic is cheaper either. Glass sounds like a good idea but do you know how long an oil would have to sit in a bottle to begin absorbing anything from it's bottle? Years.

TIP: Gas.... It's all about indigestion. Gas forming organisms in your gastro-intestinal tract are only alive because of an alkaline environment. If you add a little acid, they die. This is why I eat cabbage products like Sauerkraut, which ferment in the intestines, producing lactic acid and balances the pH of the rectum. That's a good thing.

So all things considered, eat your vegetables, like them or not. I have low fat sausage with my Sauerkraut...

If you do not like vegetables, start with one bite this week, and two bites next week, three the following until a full serving is possible. This applies to those of you with irritable bowel too. You MUST.

FOOD GROUP #8 – FIBROUS GARDEN VEGETABLES

Parts of all vegetables you purchase are dead. The natural enzymes that are in them have already caused many of their important parts it to visibly decay. At least 25% of the vital nutrients are missing from the freshest of our foods and it would be smart to take a supplement to replace them. Fresh or frozen, these treats are valuable sources of many things including fibrous bulk or "FIBER" which keeps everything sliding through your intestines smoothly. This is important because if the backside is clogged up, the rest of the process isn't going to function correctly either.

Fibrous vegetables do contain some carbs but these carb sources are not digested like starches. While counted in your calories, they are not significant. A pound of veggies yield around 2 or 3 grams of protein, 5 or 6 carbohydrates and about 30 calories per 4 oz. That's 100 calories or so compared to 300 or 500 calories a pound for starchy carbs like grains, potatoes or legumes. Every body needs more fiber in their diet and green plants not only provide them but also can actually be eaten with every meal so there is no excuse to avoid them. I mean this.

Garden vegetables are usually very low in carbohydrates and calories so they fit well with anything. But at LEAST eat them with the protein and fat meals. They truly are a must to enhance digestion. Vegetables come in a variety of different vehicles, each containing different nutrient profiles although they have the same calories for the most part. They come yellow, red, green, and orange in color. There's so many and I use as 5 or 6 of them at a time in salads! I do however save the starchier vegetables for carb meals instead of having them in protein salads.

We regularly head out for salads with salmon, chicken, turkey, ham, eggs, cheddar cheese, feta cheese, bleu cheese, olives, romaine lettuce, spring greens, mushrooms… You get the picture... Vegetables contain things that assist us in the efficient use of many of the other nutrients we eat and these things actually fight disease. These beneficial plant chemicals are called 'phyto-nutrients' and 'botanical factors'. That's why pills and multi-vitamins aren't good alone and you should take supplements with meals. No matter the quality or content (of which mine are the foremost), supplements still lack what's in food to allow them to assimilate: PHYTO-NUTRIENTS.

The fibrous veggies that go with protein and fat meals are sprouts, celery, endives, collards, spinach, chard, okra, herbs, kale, leeks, mushrooms, asparagus, lettuces like bibb or watercress (not iceberg however), cabbages (green and red), onions, seaweeds, radishes, mustard greens, cucumbers... Wow. That's a lot, and just examples. I think you get the idea. You can have all of the above with starches too. You can also have roots (like carrots, squashes), rutabaga, zucchinis, beets, different escarole, artichokes, cauliflower, eggplants, and turnips with your starches.... Just not with your proteins... Because these foods ARE starches... Low calorie sources, yes, but starches nonetheless.

You need the fiber to bind with even the tiniest amount of cholesterol so it can be used efficiently. Cholesterol has to be bound in order to cross the intestine lining and circulate back successfully to the liver to regulate your hormones and such. My favorite: Spinach, fried on medium heat in garlic, peppers and olive oil! Italian greens are GREAT as long as you do not add the beans to them! Some chicken marsala prepared correctly alongside those greens and I am in Heaven!

THE 12 FOOD GROUPS: CARBOHYDRATE MEALS

CARBOHYDRATE foods naturally come almost always 'fat free' in nature, which is obviously how the human body was designed to digest them. But read all labels, especially the ingredient lists. Carb foods can contain some evil stuff in them. A banana is a banana but pastas, instant potatoes, seasoned rices, and snack foods are all processed foods with chemicals in them. Carbs have within them nutrients that you'll never receive via fats or proteins, so you should eat them, but only the cleanest of selections are recommended.

Many vegetables contain phyto-estrogens, which can affect the body's healthy estrogen levels. Some are good; some are bad. Most vegetables heal you but some have been commercially altered and harm you. Beer contains estrogen too but what beer does to you is completely different than what vegetables do for you. While veggies aren't alcohols and all foods we eat are eventually turned into alcohols, when we drink an alcoholic beverage, it skips a natural biochemical process within all of us and that's the real problem. So, beer is out. And so are sugars. Don't have them. For one, make sure you aren't having healthy, fibrous carb sources mixed with extra (hidden) SUGARS.

Juices that contain corn syrup need to be eliminated entirely from your diet. NO Gator-aid or Kool-aid is allowed. NO breading, ketchup, sauces, etc. It all adds up to be extra sugar somewhere along the line that you do not need. So, watch out. Those of you on high protein plans, you can stick with what you learned up to this point. No sweat. But those of you not making the progress you're seeking, read on. I simply suggest you add a carbohydrate meal after each weight training session. But you don't have to. As long as you follow the 3 to 1 rule, you should get by without complication. Just realize your health depends upon these decisions.

While a 'reduced' carb diet does stimulate fat loss, a no-carb diet is NOT the ticket to success. The average person, male or female, naturally stores 100 to 300 essential grams of carbohydrates inside their bodies, depending on their size and muscularity. Where in the body? Some carbohydrate is always in the blood stream, 1/4 is in the liver and the rest is in your muscle. That's anywhere from 400 to in some cases, 1200 calories of carbs stored within us at any one time. That's technically enough to go without food for a day if necessary. But this carb supply (known as glycogen) depletes when we exercise and it needs replaced. If it isn't, our muscles are turned into sugar to save the organs from being broken down.

It is not a fat burning process that we experience when we are low on carbs. It is ketosis. The burning of ketones which come from amino acids (proteins, muscle) NOT fat... So, we at least need to replace carbs lost from exercise to preserve muscle tissue. Having a carb meal after training is a step in the right direction and 2 carb meals a day will satisfy most all of us. I am dead serious about your eating carbs separate from proteins and fats. Starches, as essential and healthy as they are, can be as bad as any other sugar if eaten with fats and proteins.

That is, unless of course, it is naturally found within the protein or fat source itself like with nuts or seeds. NEVER add starches to a fat or protein source on your own. If a food contains all three macro-nutrients at once (carbs, fats, proteins), you can still eat it, but have it separate from any other foods. In most cases, there isn't a worry in minimal amounts, like slivered almonds on your chicken. But if you're literally pouring it on, STOP. How do you determine what is low fat enough of a carb food? Multiply the total fat grams by 9 and divide that number by the total calories. If it isn't less than 10%, don't eat it.

FOOD GROUP #9 – BEANS AND LEGUMES

Beans are something vegetarians think are protein sources but they are not a substantial protein source. They are however a grand source of complex fibers known as fructo-oligo saccharides. These fibers contain a bulk which humans do not digest, but use it as nourishment of healthy bacteria in our bowels. Baked beans have a bad reputation for giving you gas but it is only due to the bacon and sugar you load on them, not because you ate them alone. If you eat beans regularly by themselves, gas will eventually disappear into thin air.... Without odor…

Examples of good legume selections are lima, pinto, kidney, lentil, black, chick, garbanzo, navy, cow, fava, red, butter beans, or blackeye peas... Every type of bean except string green and wax beans are complex starchy carb sources. Green and wax beans are low in carbohydrate, high in fiber and are better suited for one of the upcoming 12 Food Groups. The same goes with peas and corn. Most people consider them grains, but they fall more closely in line with the nourishment provided by legumes.

Beans (peas and corn too) contain approximately 75 calories, 4 grams of protein and 15 carbohydrates per 4 ounces (oz). How do I eat beans? I will make my own from dehydrated or I will eat frozen and I sometimes have canned but I never eat beans, which are packed or stored in sugars or corn syrups. Once I have read the labels to be sure, I will mix salsa with peas and black beans... I often make navy beans with fat free dumplings... I also love my rice and red beans with Cajun spices.... And I make a 4 bean chili that most chefs would envy... Peas, black beans and salsa or corn and peppers… All good mixes… As long as all items from Food Groups 1 through 7 are kept away from them...

FOOD GROUP #10 – BREADS, CEREALS, AND GRAINS

Grains are high quality starchy carbohydrates that contain soluble fiber and come from the likes of brown or wild rice, flours such as, barley, millet (which is a non-gluten grain), rye, wheat, pumpernickel, oats, and bulgur which are all used to make cereals, breads, and such. Grains are really most anything that's a tan-like pasta, or pancakes but NOT beer. Remember, beer contains hops, which contain estrogen, which is something that causes fat cells to expand. Abstain from beer if you have a 'beer belly.' If it don't look good, you don't look good!

Snacks like fig newtons, muffins, cakes and others are all A-OK if they are truly made from whole grains and contain no added sugars or fats. As far as what I eat, I eat whole grains (outer bran, inner endosperm and sprouting germ all intact) and avoid processed products as much as possible. For instance, let's look at wheat. Wheat starts off as a berry. It looks like a grain of rice and is then broken down in a milling process under a roller. The germ, the bran and the carbohydrates are all separated this way. The carbohydrates inside are then pulverized into flour (eventually bleached white), but the germ (the brown part, containing the oil and vitamin E) and bran (containing the B-vitamins) are thrown aside.

What do they do with it all? Pigs are fed the germ, cows are fed the bran, and we humans are left with white useless filling. That is the problem with refined flour. The nutrients are gone and it is virtually useless. Whole grains and cereals are GREAT for you and generally contain 4 grams of protein, 20 carbohydrates, and 1 gram of fat per 100 calories or so. Many flours are merely colored to look 'whole' grain... Always read your food labels first to be certain what you are getting into checking for added fats or sugars. I cannot repeat that statement often enough.

FOOD GROUP #11 – POTATOES

Contain both starches and sugary carbohydrates. All types of potatoes or 'tubers' (including pumpkin) are rich in the very powerful healer, potassium chloride, so even if it's just once in a while, work them into your diet. Red, yellow, baking, sweet, yam, purple, Yukon... Nothing beats a baked potato topped with nonfat butter, onions and nonfat soy bacon flavored bits or a yam with cinnamon and nonfat cream! Mmmmm!

Something the size of a medium potato (3 oz.) should have around 3 grams of protein, 22 carbohydrates and 100 calories. Although they contain both starch and sugars, these are natural sugars and a healthy combo in this case. Again, the key is no ADDED sugar... One of my treats is sliced potatoes sprinkled with sea salt and baked in the oven. I dip them in no sugar added tomato sauce. During the holidays I make stuffing without added fat, mix in peas, mushrooms and bake not only a yam, but a sweet potato for one of my meals. Alright, I lied. I eat this same meal 3 or 4 times on Holidays!

My ham, turkey and prime rib (our holiday meats) are eaten with fresh broccoli dipped in garlic butter. Vegans, just so you're not left out, I also love those 'fake' turkey dinners available at most health food stores. I guess I've just admitted to eating like a horse on holidays too. The differences are that I do not mix the foods or meals incorrectly, I do not pass out after over eating and I am not anywhere near overweight as a result of eating properly the rest of the time.

The only potato I do not like is the couch potato. I think there is no excuse for someone who has all the time in the world to sit around and do nothing all day due to their lack of attention to their eating habits or failing to exercise for 20 minutes 3 days a week...

FOOD GROUP #12 – FRUITS AND JUICES

These are sweet and sugary sources of carbohydrates that are to be eaten only during AM hours and as a dessert of sorts, following most everything else. After a carbohydrate meal or all alone by themselves, they are most enjoyable, I personally think. If you are healthy and have your body fat under control, an all fruit, no added sugar jelly or jam is wonderful on toast, bagels, etc. Berries in my cereal are great too. But again, if you haven't been eating right, have dug yourself a nice, deep hole of belly aches through poor nutrition, then you may want to have fruit alone for a while.

Sweet grapes, apples, mangoes, kiwis, applesauce, figs (did you know every fig has a bug in it), plums, papayas, nectarines, plantain bananas, dates, raisins, cherries, pears, honeydew, cantaloupe and prunes, just to name a few (prunes increase intestinal contractions and bowel fluid secretion like phenolphthalein, the chemical used in many laxatives) are all fantastic in maintaining your digestive health. Potatoes and tomatoes are actually considered 'almost' fruits too you know! But these fruits aren't the same as acidic fruits.

The acidic fruits are oranges, grapefruits, pineapples, tomatoes, lemons, limes, peaches (actually peaches and tomatoes are low carbohydrate fruits), sour apples, sour pears, apricots, berries, and sour grapes… Sour things. Think tart. Like sweet fruits, sour ones should also be eaten after a meal, by themselves, and completely separate from sweet fruits and starches, if you have digestive issues. Eating acids with starches destroys the enzymes that digest those starches. That's why we also shouldn't have vinegar on grains, potatoes, beans... 4 ounces of fruit or a piece the size of a medium banana has 24 grams of carbohydrates and 100 calories or so.

Have fruit, but do not live off of it. You know, fruits are most commonly associated with cakes, pies, desserts, creams... And there is a reason they are used in such sinful pleasures. They are high in sugar. Fruits contain essential nutrients no other foods supply but we do not need 10 bananas a day to receive them. You can have a couple pieces a day if you like, but making fruits the staple source of carbohydrates in your plan is only going to backfire on you. What about juicing?

Well, if you do drink juices, they should always absolutely be the last things you ingest after a carbohydrate meal ONLY (post workout maybe). Yes, I have heard it all before too. Drinking juices during a fast may relax your digestive system but they do not contain as much nourishment as the pulp left behind to produce them does. I do not care what nonsense you heard on TV from that crazy old guy with the bushy eyebrows. The magic of nature comes from eating whole foods, not raping them of their virtue. Natural sugars like pure maple syrup have a healing effect on the liver after it has emptied itself out all night long and depleted itself of glycogen. Blackstrap molasses works well at this too.

Having a tablespoon in my water upon waking is the closest you'll catch me at adding sugars to my diet. A glass of juice, around 8 ounces, has close to 120 calories and it's 30 grams of just plain old plant sugar. If you are drinking store bought juices, make sure it does not contain any added sugars similar to 'glucose solids' or 'corn syrup' at least. You'll overload your pancreas and make yourself FAT thinking it's healthy regardless of how healthy you think your selections are. Wine? One glass, every other day, mid-evening, after dinner is fine. But no more than that. If you want to argue the matter, you're a drunk. Just kidding.

But do us both a favor; never drink to a point of intoxication. Soda? Please. Burping after a fine swig is enough proof the body is rejecting it so get a clue. Glycemic index ratings, typically used by diabetics to gauge the rate their foods burn once eaten, are thrown in our faces more than they should be and are easily summed up. This 'index' is only important to people who eat junk food. The 12 Food Groups puts things into enough perspective for anyone to straighten their blood sugar levels out. Eat real food as often as you can and avoid processed foods. Period.

So rather than worry about the glycemic index or eating one food over another because you are a diabetic, make sure you have several forms of carbs at a time or at least have them separate from your proteins and fats. For instance, if you have a banana, have a banana and a whole grain bagel. If you have pasta, have sauce and veggies. If you have rice, have soy sauce and beans too.

I had a 235 pound 65 year old lady come to me once. She had been an insulin dependent diabetic for 50 years at that point. 2 months later, she was down to 205 and her doctor told us she no longer needed well over half of her insulin. She still fought me tooth and nail over the diet and ate twice what I asked her. This went on throughout our relationship. Yet, despite her convictions, the end result was still success. The 12 Food Groups WORK. She dropped 45 pounds of fat and gained 15 pounds of muscle during that time.

I can't tell you how many women I have encountered or that have emailed me who are guilty of eating just fruit all day in an effort to lose weight. Success is achieved by having combinations of the 12 Food Groups, not by enjoying only one group a day.

SIMPLE CALORIE COUNTING TIPS

1) Eggs: A larger whole egg (white and yolk together) contains about 6 grams of protein, 4 grams of fat and 60 calories. The white alone has 5 grams of protein and 20 calories and the yolk has 1 gram of protein and all the fat.

2) Seafood: Averages 23 grams of protein and 3 grams of fat per quarter pound (4 ounces).

3) Animal meats: Trimmed of visible fat and skin, contain on the average quarter (1/4) pound, almost 25 grams of protein, 5 grams of fat and 135 calories.

4) Organ meats: On the average, 1/3 pound or 5 1/3 ounces contain 20 grams of protein, 10 grams of fat and 170 calories.

5) Dairy products: Low fat cheeses have around 8 grams of protein, 1 or 2 carbohydrates, 5 grams of fat, and about 80-85 calories an ounce. Non-fat milk and yogurts are about 8 grams of protein and 12 to 16 carbohydrates per 8 ounces.

6) Nuts and seeds: An ounce (1 oz.) of seeds, nuts or nut butter contains around 7 grams of protein, 7 carbohydrates, 14 grams of fat and 182 calories. Some are higher or lower in these figures.

7) Fats and oils: A tablespoon of oil contains almost 14 grams of fat and 126 calories. Get your essential fatty acid oil from www.lemmonsoil.com

8) Fibrous Garden Vegetables: Veggies yield around 2 or 3 grams of protein, 5 or 6 carbohydrates and around 30 calories per 4 oz.

9) Beans (legumes): Approximately 75 calories, 4 grams of protein and 15 carbohydrates per 4 ounces (oz). That's one fourth of a 16 oz can.

10) Grains: Grains and cereals generally contain 4 grams of protein, 20 carbohydrates, and 1 gram of fat per 110 calories.

11) Potatoes: Something the size of a medium potato (3 oz.) should have around 3 grams of protein, 22 carbohydrates and 100 calories.

12) Fruits: 4 ounces or a piece the size of a good banana has 24 grams of carbohydrates and 100 calories more or less. Medium sized apples are usually 3 oz and contain 80 calories.

MEASUREMENTS THAT REALLY MATTER..

Calves: Stand feet together, all weight shifted off the leg being measured. Relax. Wrap the tape around the thickest part.

Today: [ ]   Again in 13 Weeks: [ ]

Thighs: Measure both of them. Spread your feet about six inches apart and shift your weight to the leg not being measured. Be completely relaxed and tape the largest part. Don't be shy.

Today: [ ]   Again in 13 Weeks: [ ]

Buttocks: Stand up straight, feet flat, relaxed, heels together. Measure around the (gulp) biggest part off your caboose!

Today: [ ]   Again in 13 Weeks: [ ]

Hips: Same position. Keep standing. Measure just a little higher than the butt. I know, I don't like it either… Just do it…

Today: [ ]   Again in 13 Weeks: [ ]

Waist: Place the tape one inch above the belly button or around the largest part. Measure from the back and ['don't' ?]close your eyes!

Today: [ ]   Again in 13 Weeks: [ ]

Chest: Lift your arms out to the side at shoulder height and wrap the tape under your armpits. Let your arms come down again and relax.

The measurer should tape you right across the nipples all the way around. We aren't measuring lung capacity so don't take in a deep breath. Ladies, you know what to do here.

Today: [ ]   Again in 13 Weeks: [ ]

Shoulders: Tape around the widest part. Again, relax...

Today: [ ]   Again in 13 Weeks: [ ]

Upper Arms: Raise the arm to be measured straight out to the side palms up and keep it relaxed. Measure where it appears to be thickest and then do the same spot on the other arm too.

Today: [ ]   Again in 13 Weeks: [ ]

Forearms: Out of curiosity, go ahead and measure your forearms while you have your arm extended.

Today: [ ]   Again in 13 Weeks: [ ]

Body Weight: No one wants to admit they weigh more or than they consider optimal but get on that scale now! It's IMPORTANT!

Today: [ ]   Again in 13 Weeks: [ ]

BODY FAT PERCENTAGES

Before you workout or do anything else today, including the reading of this chapter, your next step in getting up off your butt and doing something about looking and feeling better is to record those tape measurements. Yes the ones I just listed. See how big your various body parts are. Get your tape out, measure your parts then let's continue. This section of this book tells you how to use that simple tape measure for a VERY accurate means by which to determine your EXACT daily caloric intake needs. After thousands of clients, it's right on the target every single time. It's not how fat or built you are that determines your caloric intake. It is your lean body mass.

So make sure that part is right first. Then forget what you think you know. This isn't as simple as your weight multiplied by 10 or 15 or 20 or whatever either. It seems that many people believe the thyroid gland is a major key in fat loss. It may be, but it's what you do to the rest of your body that affects your thyroid and fat loss most. People also think dieting slows the metabolism and therefore the thyroid down. Others believe the marketing and seek the use of caffeine pills (diet pills of any sort) as their obvious solution.

Others believe surgeons who say if you are too fat or too thin, you should have your thyroid removed. The truth is, fat people have slow thyroids because they allowed themselves to get fat. Thin people do not have fast thyroids, they have poor eating habits as well. A fat person who becomes thin will find that their otherwise slow thyroid suddenly returned to normal after they lost the extra weight. Skinny people who begin eating better, put on a little muscle only to find that their thyroids have regulated too. You do the math. Dietary habits interfere with the metabolism and slow the function of your thyroid.

Weight problems are not caused by the thyroid gland initially not working right. Weight problems are caused over time by YOU to a point your organs fail. Face it. YOU 'made' YOU over or under weight. YOU also make yourself unhealthy. Overweight people tell me all the time that they eat less often than you think they do. They usually eat like a pig once a day, usually only at night, and starve themselves all day long. You know that's not good. Underweight people eat all the time but rarely do they eat enough, and that's their problem. Look, I had two sisters come in to my office both weighing 160 pounds.

They also each had 25% body fat which means they had about 120 pounds of muscle mass and 40 pounds of body fat apiece. They were twins and both told me they were to begin thyroid medication in 28 days as prescribed by their physician. Have you ever dieted but only got fatter? Listen to this then… One sister ignored my recommendations because she thought 'my' plan was nonsense. She didn't agree with giving up sweets, sodas, nor McDonald's French fries. She felt that protein powder was more important than fresh proteins, vegetables, grains, etc. She lost weight and went from 160 to 130 in 28 days.

The problem was, all her weight lost was in muscle. She now had 90 pounds of muscle (down 30) and 40 pounds of body fat (the same as where she started) at the 130 pounds she now weighed. This had her now at 31.77% body fat instead of the 25% she started off at! She looked AWFUL too. Truly obese and disgusting with all that loose skin and cellulite. Got cellulite? That is due to eating both table and fake sugars (chewing gum and drinking soda), not eating enough essential fats, nor drinking enough water. All the things she kept doing. Her sister on the other hand listened to what I had to say and although she only lost 20 pounds, it was all in fat.

It doesn't matter if she lost ALL the weight she wanted to, it matters that she did the right thing, she LOOKED REALLY GOOD and SHE GOT REALLY HEALTHY doing it. Going from 160 to 140 brought her body fat down from 25% to 14.3% (as opposed to the 31.77% her sister achieved by starving herself)! One of them was told by their physician not to start taking thyroid medicine. Guess which one... I will save the weight gain stories for another chapter. What you are about to read next will become the blueprint for everything you do regarding food intake for the rest of your life. Take it very seriously. Take your body fat percentage very seriously.

The International Sports Sciences Association says 5% of your total body weight being fat for men, and 8% for women is the minimum you need to sustain a healthy body. Are you anywhere near that low? They also say 10% for men and for women 15% is optimal (which I whole heartedly agree) and anything above 20% for men, or 25% for women is, I am sorry, just plain unacceptable. That's clinical obesity. Chronic obesity is anything above 25% for men and 30% for women.

Not much of a difference really. By the time you are above 20% fat, you're already worrying about what others think. I am sorry if you are in this group, I feel your pain, but please, do not turn back now. I am here for you. However, I want you to know the facts no matter how painful they are to hear. 15% for men and 20% for women may be comfortable for some, but as a whole, society has either made us far too comfortable with being fat. We are generally confused about how lean we really ought to become. Let's stick with 10% for men and 15% for the ladies.

This will get you to the beach without wearing dresses or t-shirts the entire time. How much body fat DO YOU have? Maybe you should get a professional body fat analysis performed and find out. In fact, have two or three done and "average" out the results. They shouldn't be more than $20 a pop. If they are, you can get skin-fold calipers instead, but that's not fast enough. We need to get started today. So instead of thumbing through the phone book to see if someone in your area uses

"Bio- Impediance" body fat (composition) equipment or professional skin-fold calipers (calipers measure pinches of body fat all over you to determine fat levels), let's act quick. What I need you to do right now is take 3 'before and after' pictures. Go ahead, grab a camera. Stand like a crucifix with your arms out to the sides and up at shoulder height.

Have someone take a picture from the front, from the side and one from the back. Make sure you are at least in the picture from your ankles to the top of your head. We need to see what you are made of, so wear revealing clothing, don't cover up. We will use these photos as 'before' and 'after' progress reports to 'witness' your progress. Take them by standing in front of a white wall wearing fat revealing clothing like short shorts and either no shirt or a sports bra (ladies are the only ones supposed to wear a bra or bikini top, yes, some jokers have sent me silly stuff in the past). BUT JUST DO IT. After all, you will never look like this again!

Embarrassed or not, you need proof! Later down the road, when you are being re-measured, photographed, weighed or whatever, continue to use the same scale, tape measure, camera, equipment or technician in order to maintain the integrity of your results. Deal? Ok... Do you know how much body fat you have right now but aren't being honest with us? Forget about scheduling a body fat test, we haven't that sort of time. If you do know your body fat %, great, if not, we'll simply use your waist measure.

With some of you, I realize that you may or may not have a lot of fat around your waist right now. You may be trying to gain weight instead of losing it too. I still want you to measure your waist for me. Is it what you want it to be? For every inch bigger than it is supposed to be, you have a good 5 to 7 pounds of fat to lose. For instance, let's say there are 6 extra inches around your belly (or BUTT, if you store the fat in your hips and booty, measure that instead...).

Ladies, 6 inches of unwanted flubber is a good 30 pounds you need to lose in body fat for sure. It could be more, it could be less, but it's close. You know whether you are too fat or not without measuring but measuring the fattest part of your body, also gives us approximately about how much lean mass you have.

Knowing this information will give us a good indication of what your minimum daily caloric intake should be too. Confused? Forget about it! Fill out the following info.

1. Your Current Body Weight Is:
2. Your Current Waist Measure Is:
3. The Most Realistic Waist Measure For You Is:
4. The Difference Between The Two Measures Are:
5. Multiply The Difference By 6:
6. Deduct The Above Figure From Actual Weight:
7. Divide Step 6's Result By Ten (10):
8. Multiply Step 6's Result By Step 7's Result:
Step 8's Result Is Your Daily Calorie Recommendation.

Next...
1. Divide Results Of Step 6 By Your Body Weight:
2. Subtract The Above Result From 1.000:
3. Multiply The Above By 100. Your Body Fat % Is:

HAVING SIX MEALS A DAY

Realize the caloric figure you come up with may seem higher than you have been eating OR it may be even lower. It is easy to recommend a fixed amount of calories (also known as energy) for anyone using this formula. This represents an estimate of what you need to survive efficiently each day on. Whatever you're doing now, adjust your calories to be closer to what we have come up with right here. It's important you do this.

Now that you know how many calories you are supposed to consume, divide those calories by 6. It is best for you to have the same amount of calories at each feeding right now, and six is the minimum number of meals you should be having each day. I know, "How could I possibly fit six meals into MY schedule?" Easy. Breakfast, Brunch, Lunch, Mid-Day Break, Dinner and Mid-Evening. If you want to or currently already eat more often than this, simply divide your daily calories by 7, 8, 9 or however many meals you plan to have each day. I often eat 10 times a day. Upon waking, on the way out the door, mid-morning, lunch, mid-day, mid-afternoon, dinner, mid-evening, before bed.... Wait. That's only 9! Well, whenever I have the time, it's alright to eat more often. Just don't OVER eat…

Eating more than 5 times a day gives you a metabolic edge over other people especially when those meals are all equal in calories. Rest assured eating 6, 7 or 8 times a day following this simple rule, you cannot become fat. There is no way on earth clean food in the right amounts can fatten anyone up especially if they follow the program every single day for even a month.

A meal every 2 hours is acceptable. Let's start right now by determining what your plans are for the next few hours. Are you at home? Are you out or heading out? Will you have time to stop for food? Should you pack a snack to take with you? What did you eat last? Should the next meal be a carb or a protein meal? Do you need both because you will be out for the next couple of feedings or the entire day? Are you going to be working out? Or will you possibly be napping soon?

Are you trying to lose weight or gain weight? Too much to think about right now? No matter what runs through your mind when you think about eating 6 times a day, know that an hour should never pass without fresh food being already in or going in to the belly and this is the single most valuable habit you can adopt. You must give the body a continuous supply of nutrients for building muscle, burning fat, keeping your energy levels up and blood sugar regulated. Face it. Your way didn't work or you wouldn't be here. I am an industry insider. I probably know something that you do not. You can't risk that I don't because odds are you only disagree because you haven't done this before. So how would you know? Trust me...

Ever had a hunger pang? Growling belly? That means the body has gone into a catabolic state because you're not eating often enough. Not good. That also means you are losing muscle, which in turn leads to the storing of more body fat. Don't like that fat on your back? Speed the metabolism... Eat something! You will notice that when you cut calories back on a typical diet you don't get hungry. This is only because you are mixing your foods the wrong way and they do not digest properly. Your meal just sits there in your gut, so you never get the signal that it's time to eat again. This is BAD.

One reason we have equal sized meals is to teach you that meals are not meant to be Holiday-sized feedings just to hold you over until you eat again but moderately sized and sensibly prepared feedings that your body can digest more easily. Keep your energy levels constant. Several medium sized portions a day digest easily. Eating small meals one at a time adds up to more and more food by the day's end, which is better than eating everything all at once. There is no starving and no letting the metabolic fires from within slow down on you. This is key.

Only eating one or two large meals to make up for your supposedly cramped schedule is unacceptable. Look where you are. You're not in your best shape. Admit it. We can all fit 6 feedings in if we WANT to... Let's move on. So, with that said, breakfast, lunch and dinner are not going to be enough to elicit the results even if you eat from all 'four' food groups and take your wonder supplements bought off the television. We need food and nourishment all day long, especially in the morning, so let's begin there.

Breakfast is usually skipped because people don't feel like eating or think they haven't time. Well, if you do not eat breakfast (especially before working out or within 10 minutes of waking, the body shuts things off inside of you to prevent excessive muscle or organ loss. This is the first thing you're doing wrong that leads to fat storage. When we starve, the body's priority is to protect your insides from eating away at themselves for the energy that they are not getting from food. Food, we can all agree, is what we were designed to run off, not out, of anyhow.

That's why we crave the stuff, get rumbles in the tummy and why I repeat it again and again so you will remember it. Without food, the body cannot do the things you want it to yet run efficiently... Let's assume then we were actually created to get our nourishment by leaching specific nutrients little by little from the foods we ingest. Foods are, for the most part, made up of carbohydrates, proteins and/or fats that happen to contain all the essential vitamins, minerals, amino and fatty acids you require for EVERY SINGLE HUMAN FUNCTION there is. This is stuff we all understand. It is also common sense that if you want fully nourished, you MUST try to eat all sorts of different foods at some point during each day.

Foods do not always provide what we need however. This is

why we must add certain supplements to the diet. We can also surmise that in order to get enough of the essential nutrients, we would be required to ingest more food than we have time for too. Sure, I bet some of you already do eat six times a day but having bird-sized meals followed up by feasts doesn't count for much in this scenario. If you aren't 100% completely certain you have control over how much, what time, and what specific foods you eat at one meal opposed to another, you had better become so today. We need carbs, fats and proteins just to make it through a day. The sources of those nutrients may vary. On occasion, what we think is nourishing us is really leaching from us or feeding the toxins that make us tired, sick and fat.

I cannot twist your arm to eat more food and to do so more often. You are correct about that. However, oddly enough, without enough calories there aren't enough 'macro' nutrients (carbs, fats, proteins) so all your expensive supplements, which hopefully contain all 'micro' or 'trace' nutrients, are most often useless. When I first began eating right, I hadn't any idea eating the correct amount of food each day would make a difference either. I would wake up, eat a box of cereal, chug a gallon of milk, boil a pound of pasta, eat 3 pounds of fish, and by the end of the first few days always ended up quitting because I only got fat in the process. After that, I would panic and eat only a can of tuna the first 3 meals of the day then wonder why I was losing muscle. So yes, I know what a yo-yo diet can do to your appearance first hand.

Do you experience any of the following after eating: Mental grogginess? Yawning? Falling asleep in class or at work? Thoughts begin to cloud? Choose your words wrong? Nasal congestion? Hives? Belching? Well, times are about to change.

Now you're listening? Well, I've got another story for you...

CARB MEALS VS. PROTEINS AND FATS

Like an automobile, does it make sense to try and drive without gasoline, oil or transmission fluid in your engine? No? We agree there. Good. Then why would you insist on low quality products to run it or blindly mix gasoline and oil together into your engine at the same time? The body cannot produce the enzymes to separate fuels by itself. You need many different sorts of fuel to operate a car, but a car doesn't store each component in the same areas, nor can it separate them to save its parts if you mix the wrong fuels together. And if you want your body's fuels (food) to digest efficiently, you DO NOT mix them incorrectly either.

No matter how low fat, low carbohydrate, high protein, vegetarian or wholesome your eating habits are.... There are rules to be abided if you want control of your health and appearance. Besides having at least 6 meals of equal caloric intake, you must always be certain to keep carbohydrate foods away from your protein and fat foods. Carbohydrates require neither fat NOR does protein require sugar to assist in it's digestion. In fact, these nutrients inhibit one another's usage. If you eat protein with starchy carbohydrates, one goes incompletely digested.

Thus, the feeling like a basketball is sitting in your gut after you eat them together (like a cheese burger). The myth that you need carbs and protein together for additional glucose in your blood to transport the digested amino acids is unfounded. Most of the sugar used to transport protein comes from previously eaten carbohydrates, not from what's eaten at that particular meal! Carbs spare your amino acids and proteins from being used as energy, only if you eat them separately. Otherwise, protein doesn't get used efficiently at all.

Sure, most all carbs have some protein in them. However, the protein that nature provides in a fruit, vegetable or grain does not have the same biological composition of meat or fish protein. It's obvious there is a chemical difference between an egg and oatmeal or they would be the same thing. One is from a plant, the other is from an animal. With that said, keep your proteins and fats together and clear of added starchy carbohydrates. Fat plays a major role in hormone production but only ends up wasted when eaten with carbs. Contained in all protein foods, like meat and eggs, there is always a little natural fat in whatever we choose to eat.

As mentioned in the 12 Food Groups chapter, you should trim the skin off the meats you eat, toss aside the marbled fat, then add healthy fat back to your meal... Protein naturally requires fat to assist in its digestion, and that's why all protein sources in natural forms do contain fat, but the skin unfortunately isn't the best source of quality nutrients. Not interested in hearing that? Who do you know on a low fat diet that is not doing so well? If you eat no fat, the result is always poor hormone levels. That means little to no muscle growth for men, difficult menstrual cycles and blotchy skin for women and very little fat loss for every body. Signs of protein deficiency.

And so you know, protein with a little fat eaten a couple hours before bed will increase your natural secretion of growth hormone in response to a decreased blood sugar level that occurs naturally as you enter into sleep. So eating late at night is 'good' for you after all... That is if you ate SIX meals the same day beforehand... Many of my top models and bodybuilders do this... I know what you're thinking, but there really isn't a comparison to eating right and having a plate of spaghetti and meatballs before sleep...

DIGESTION REQUIRES ATTENTION

Did you know that you could take a pill with different enzymes to break down different foods, depending on what you wanted to eat? Well, the body does this for you. The enzymes that act upon carbohydrates are not the ones that act upon proteins and fats and vice versa. The pharmacies who make your over the counter enzymes know this, your doctor knows this, but for some reason, no one told you to eat accordingly. Instead, they simply made a pill available. Taking digestive enzymes with your meals is like admitting you are doing something wrong, but you aren't sure what. It's nothing more than a band-aid, which you can swallow. Is that natural? No. Am I sure of this?

Yes, I am 100% absolutely sure that carbohydrates require different enzymes than protein. Look up alpha amylase, sucrase, etc. which all break down carbs and then look into the various peptidases for protein like trypsin and chymotripsin, you'll see what the truth is for yourself. One thing is for sure, you'll discover that metabolisms are completely separate and different for these different foods. It is very possible you went to school or have researched this before but haven't seen anything to indicate that only one set of enzymes or another can be released at a time in your belly. You either overlooked it or depended upon whatever your trainer or favorite magazine said instead of looking it up on your own. Research it again.

It'll be right there in front of you. Trial and error, along with actual footwork, takes a person a long way. My path led me to the conclusion we were made this way intentionally. I haven't a clue why we were created to digest food like this but it seems most religions agree, food was made for man, not man for the food.

So, I am pretty certain the Creator designed our bodies to digest what was prepared for us. And even if not, we can at least agree that plants and animals, while both contain life, are completely different things. Almost any medical doctor will admit, carbohydrates require a completely different metabolism and set of enzymes to digest than proteins do. Ask one. They should be able to at least confirm that the release of hydrochloric acid (in the stomach) lowers pH to a level (below 3.5), which inactivates alpha-amylase (one of the enzymes which break down carbohydrates) to allow protein to better digest.

This alone lends credibility to my program. If they can't, they either haven't paid attention to their nutrition and digestion or as I said, they possibly overlooked it. An obvious sign your foods aren't digesting properly is GAS. Agree? Well, just bear with me, follow the program and if after 30 days on the Know How the gas is GONE, then it's safe to assume with those results you are making some sort of progress. Right?

Upon chewing the first bite of food at breakfast, the necessary enzymes to break down your food of choice are secreted and become present in the gut all based upon what the food is recognized as by the brain. Once this meal is eaten, it pushes whatever is left in the belly from the previously eaten 'last' meal, meat for instance, through the duodenum into the small intestine. Other enzymes are then secreted (like tyrosine and chymotrypsin) in order to deal with scavenging your previously digested mush for amino acids and fats. This is why you shouldn't skip breakfast even if you're not hungry. The lack of hunger comes from food still being in the gut. It needs moved out so the body can do it's job correctly. No, this isn't when you poop it out, but it determines whether your metabolism is up to par.

Metabolism is the process where cells either create through anabolism or destroy through catabolism. Catabolism is the process of living tissue being broken down and turned into energy or waste. This is destructive. Anabolism is the process of construction. You want the body as anabolic as possible to burn fat, build and maintain muscle and speed the metabolism… So keep eating… Because of breakfast, that protein meal that you ate last night is now pushed into the small intestine and is being absorbed into the blood stream. Amino acids from that food are being distributed throughout the body to build and repair tissue (this is what is meant by maintaining a positive nitrogen balance when dealing in protein metabolism). But that's not all.

This process of getting breakfast in, so the remnants of last night's meal goes down, also pushes yet another meal from the day before, into the large intestine. The process of pushing the food all the way through requires yet another meal because you can store two or three meals in your backside at any given time. Most studies done on digestion were performed using people eating a variety of foods together, not separate. This is why they say the basic reality boils down to carbs digesting faster than proteins, which digest faster than fats. That's true, but that's from mixing foods and giving the body no other choice and why it takes a 'normal' meal 6 hours to leave the stomach unless you put something on top of it to push it through.

If for no other reason and to avoid constipation, PLEASE do not skip meals no matter what happens. If you feel you won't be able to eat on time, eat sooner, never later. Skipping meals leaves food inside of you to rot. That's not good. If you do not listen to your body, food can sit in your digestive tract long enough that it actually begins to spoil.

This is part of the reason you stink so much when you break wind or eventually do go to the bathroom. Stinky, putrid food has been clogging up your digestive tract. You receive little or none of the nutrients you are expecting to from letting this happen. They will die in there before ever getting to be absorbed if you do not eat in a timely fashion. Remember, the stomach is merely the first stop. That same food must somehow next exit the gut and enter the intestines to begin nourishing you. Not only is it a waste if the food cannot continue this simple trek, but the spoiling process is what creates the toxins that make you sick, tired, stinky and slows your metabolism down.

Sad thing is, it really is such a simple and easy process to assist along. You just have to eat another meal. If not, it will be the accumulated toxins from years of bad eating habits that slowly and quietly poison you to death. Ever heard this story before? "But Joe was just over to the house last week. He didn't have cancer." YES, he did. It wasn't found in time because not only wasn't he getting checkups but these things catch up to you. Once they do, you're in trouble seemingly over night. It's too late now for Joe. You however can make change NOW.

He's dead at age 38 from colon cancer. Are you ready to extend your life or did you want to go pick out your coffins and head-stone instead? It's that serious. All that fat, saggy, blotchy skin, and lack of muscle means inside, you are dying. Literally dying. I don't care if you are 16 or 60. You're killing yourself. Wish you could be like you were when you were younger and hate what you see in the mirror, especially when you are naked? Well, do SOMETHING like EAT ON TIME. Assuming it takes 1/2 hour to finish a typical meal, and you could easily schedule your meals 3 hours apart, waiting 2 and a half hours after fin-ishing a meal is about average time to begin eating again.

If you aren't hungry this often, now you know it's because THERE'S UNDIGESTED FOOD IN YOUR GUT waiting to be pushed through. The stomach rarely empties on it's own effi-ciently. You just think it does because eventually you get hun-gry. So, humor me, just in case something doesn't get efficient-ly digested from the previous meals you ate, it is always a good idea to make sure it gets pushed through your digestive tract anyhow. Think of the food in your stomach as a clog in a sink or toilet drain. Substantial forces must be applied to move what's clogging the pipes down and out your drainage (and in this case, your digestive) system.

You'll always be 'clogged' or 'backed up' unless eat on time and ingest equally sized meals. This leads me to my next point. If you do not have bowel movements regularly, you are in more trouble than you realize. FULL bowel movements are normal if performed more than twice daily. Dropping pebble sized 'poops' do NOT count as 'going' to the bathroom. No matter what you believe causes your constipation nor whether you think it will go away on it's own, eat something. Eat something again in 2 and a half more hours. Eventually, you'll go to the bathroom regularly again. And for heaven's sake! ALWAYS chew your food slowly and thoroughly (with your mouth shut and lips together please)! Your stomach has no teeth. If you're still getting gas, that is why. Sure, there is the possibility you may be drinking too much water with your meals too, but either way, chew slowly, keep your lips closed, digest well, excrete it out, repeat...

RECAP: One meal goes in the belly. A second meal pushes it through to the small intestine. A third pushes it into the large intestine. A fourth pushes it almost out of you. If you are eating enough at those first 4 meals, it may have pushed through. If not, 5 meals should. 6 meals always does....

PROPER MEAL PLANNING

Six meals merely optimizes things so like most healthy people, you can experience a couple healthy movements a day. No, I do not mean you'll have diarrhea nor to offend you with all my poo poo talk. Understand, if food were meant to stay inside of you, there wouldn't be a means for it to come out. Nor would we be so uncomfortable when it doesn't. I used to think 3 meals were all you need. That's how I was raised. But as I got older, I craved mid evening snacks more and more often. When I began working instead of sitting around all day, if I didn't snack between meals, I couldn't function. As each meal or snack was added, the better I looked, the better I felt. Eventually a seventh meal was added and I will never eat less than that again. You can start with six…

What you should do now is determine the amount of food you are eating currently and see how it compares to those new caloric allowances we figured a few pages back using your waist measure. Take a moment and feel free to write in the book, it's yours. Try to figure up how many calories you are eating on an average day by jotting down, meal to meal what you ate today on a separate piece of paper.

Do this tomorrow if you must. Do it for the next 7 straight days too. Separate your foods, begin to eat more sensibly and take notes of everything you do from now on. Because guess what? We need to know what you're doing, how your appetite fluctuates and what your preferences are. Why? As you build muscle and eliminate fat, you will be required to eat more and more calories in order to maintain what you build and keep the results coming in. If you do not know what you are doing, how will you know what needs to be changed? Maybe you think you know... At least this way you'll be certain.

It's all about meal preparation and we are about to discuss the RIGHT way to set up a dietary road map. To start, we already know your measurements, we know your body fat percentage, we know your calorie intake and we know how many calories you need per meal. Next, we'll schedule four of your meals (or snacks) to come from the protein and fat foods we discussed in the 12 Food Groups. Metabolism is the process of every cell to either create anabolism or catabolism. It is also the process by which food is turned into useable substance by a human being. Catabolism is the process of living tissue being broken down and turned into energy and waste. This is destructive.

Do your best to eat proteins and fats at a 3 to 1 gram ratio to one another and include green vegetables. Some people think this diet has them eating less protein because we only have it 4 times a day instead of at all meals. That's not true. Because you get to eat more when you do have it, you're consuming plenty and because digestion is enhanced, more protein is actually absorbed. Not satisfied? Add a fifth meal then. But continue to have it separate from your carbs.

Others ask if 4 meals are too much. No, it is not. Take your lean mass and divide it by 3. However many pounds that is, say 180 divided by 3 is 60, then that's how many grams, 60, you should have at your 4 protein meals. Add it up at the end of a day and there is PLENTY but not too much. Divide that number of grams of protein by 3 and that is how many grams of fat should be eaten with those meals too. It's perfect. I wouldn't ask my grandfather to begin eating 240 grams a day or even the 60 grams per meal eating that much requires. But I would if he were a bodybuilder, maybe, depends on his weight. However, no matter who you are, if you eat your protein and carbs together, you might really be assimilating half of what you think you are.

With protein containing 4 calories a gram and fat having 9 calories a gram, that's 420 calories if I eat 60 grams of protein and 20 grams of fat at my protein and fat meals. I tend to have 500 calories per meal these days so adding 80 calories of say, spinach, will round my meal off perfectly. To get 60 grams of protein from nonfat cottage cheese, I will need to have a little over 2 cups which is 320 calories. This leaves me with just enough room to add 20 grams of fat from Lemmon's Oil before running out of calories. I would then just make up for not having greens by having them at another meal. Sounds like a lot of fat though doesn't it?

It really isn't when it's a healthy fat like flax seed, butter, olive or Lemmon's Oil. If I haven't convinced you to increase the fat a little, at least keep the carbs separate and maybe go with a 4 to 1 ratio instead. Do not exceed your allowed calories no matter what you decide. If you are a vegetarian, search for high quality, low carbohydrate, protein alternatives at your health food store. It's alright that you choose not to eat red meat, fish or chicken. That's fine.

I do feel eating some farm fresh eggs and organic cheese with your tofu is only going to help you in the long run. No matter the choices, round the meal off with a nice bowl of green vegetables. Next on the list, plan another two feedings as carbohydrate meals. If you do not feel like eating a lot of carbohydrates, cut back on them a little, but no matter what, always keep them separate from your protein and fat meals. Understand, you are supposed to HAVE CARBS. Limit yourself by only having two meals if you like, but do not neglect them entirely. Whatever you heard before about low carb dieting in the past, FORGET IT. It's all nonsense (for the most part) and I want you to go select items from Food Groups 8 through 12.

The hardest part of this program is reading all of the food labels of every food that you purchase before you eat it and trying to learn what the foods really are made of. Considering that any 6th grader can read a cereal box, this really shouldn't be a problem. Serving sizes DO vary quite a bit from manufacturer to manufacturer and should never be taken for granted no matter how many foods you memorize. The calorie counting at first will teach you to eat for satisfaction, not out of pleasure (gluttony). The reading of labels out of curiosity at least will make everything else seem like a piece of cake.

How many carbs are actually contained in your carb meal depends upon what foods you select. Some foods are higher or lower in protein content than others and this is what affects the amount of carbs they contain. For example, fruit doesn't really have any protein per 100 calories but a potato has around 3 grams. Beans contain 6 or 7 grams, rice 4 or 5, and some grains have up to 10 grams per 100 calories. So you see, this varies the carbohydrate contents anywhere from 15 to 25 grams depending upon what you're eating.

This is why you should always read labels. Especially if you've taken up carbohydrate counting as a second hobby... I don't want to give the impression that you have to count calories for the rest of your lives however, walking around with 4 extra inches around your gut doesn't look good. And it's not right. But by counting calories as in counting what you take in, not in limiting yourself, you will learn where to begin cutting the calories (or raising them) if necessary. You need this info so you know for certain whether you are feeding your lean muscle tissue enough to burn fat or not. But forget about limiting carbs or falling into this percentage or that percentage.

It's really not about the carbs being in a "ZONE" or below 30 grams a day that counts after all. It's about scheduling 6 meals a day and making sure 4 are protein and fat (low carb) based and that 2 are carbohydrate (low protein, low fat) based. For you Zone followers, I want you to know right now that for every pound of lean body mass you change or are different from the person next to you, there is a coinciding change in not only the amount of calories you ingest, but the basic structure of those calories and the mixtures in which you receive them! The percentages of protein, fat and carbohydrates are rarely 40-30-30 folks. Begin tallying up what you already eat and count those calories as accurately as possible if you haven't already. See if you're really in a zone at all.

This is how easy eating 6 times a day is... We all go to sleep at night at some point. We all also wake up eventually, so that's breakfast time. We all work, even if it's around the house each day, so, mid-morning, take a snack break. We are all either allowed, given or know we can take a 15 minute break. That's enough time for brunch. We all also get lunch breaks or can at least make time for one, even if it's 30 minutes later than planned. We all can. So do that too. There's 3 meals already...

Mid-day is when we all take our second shift breaks or can at least sit around long enough for a few moments to snack again. When I was a district manager of a health store chain in Los Angeles, I used to have my snacks in my car while driving. So I know you can pull it off. And I haven't met a business person yet who didn't gain the respect of his peers by making sure they took care of themselves by having a snack on time. Not one. Eventually, we all come home from work or we prepare a dinner of some sort wherever we are. We also get a craving mid-evening or sometime before bed, so eat something then too. Still not convinced? Come on, take charge for a change!

When I was in the Army, I would wake up first thing in the morning and have a glass of protein powder before heading out to do PT. After our hour-long session of pushups and running, I would go stand in line at the mess hall for an omelet and cottage cheese. On the way out, I would put bagels and bananas in my larger pants pockets to snack on and hold me over until lunch. At lunch, I ate a lot of burger meat, pork chops, cheeses and veggies. Before I left the mess hall again, I always grabbed apples and muffins for the mid-day snack. For dinner, I had more meat and veggies before cleaning up to hit the gym.

After my workout I would go to the grocery store or commissary to get a quart of nonfat milk to drink. Now of course, you can argue it isn't so easy doing this sort of thing while out in the field or playing war games in the woods. But if you're smart, and I know you are, you'll know better than that now. It's as easy as you want it to be. Another time I worked 2 jobs while studying for school. One was from 12:00 noon until 4:00 p.m. each day and the other was a 11:00 p.m. to 7:00 a.m. midnight shift. I ate at 10:30 before work, 1:00 a.m. on break, 3:30 a.m. at 'lunch' and 6:00 a.m. before the boss came in.

I would get off at 7:00, be home at 7:30 a.m. and sleep until 11:30 a.m. As soon as I would wake up, I ate and left for my second job. I ate again at 2:00 p.m. then was off work at 4:00 p.m. and back in bed from 4:30 p.m. to 6:30 p.m. I ate when I arose at 6:30 and then from 7:30 to 10:30 p.m. I was either buried in studies or going to the gym for an hour each night. Which ever it was, I ate again at 8:30 p.m. between courses or after the workout. At 10:30 the cycle started over again. Man, I needed a nap though. I was always tired.

While in the Army, I dealt with lack of sleep. If it were wartime, or if an emergency arose, you would need deal with that lack of sleep so we literally slept deprived ourselves as a form of training. But you will still 'feel' it eventually if you do not get your '8' hours of sleep each night. Sure, you can ignore the signals. But once you realize that the first 2 hours of sleep you get must be fully uninterrupted if you want your hormones to regulate and that actual healing doesn't begin until after the body has been down for 6 hours straight (and that only lasts for 2 more hours), then you might try a little harder at getting to bed EARLIER instead of LATER each night. One night with poor rest affects even the best of us for days at a time and the accumulative damage can be devastating.

In fact, in my one apartment I had this horrid cricket that seemed to like toying with me by doing all this blasted chirping only during the times I was trying to sleep! Not while anyone else slept, JUST WHILE I TRIED TO! So to ensure my 8 hours of rest, I wore earplugs. How funny is that? No, coffee and artificial stimulants will not make up for a lack of sleep. Do not use caffeine pills when you are sleep deprived unless you want ulcers later in life. And early morning isn't a good time for stimulants anyhow. As far as proper timing goes, your adrenal glands are weak in the morning but strong midday. But that isn't mid-day every-day.

You can drink coffee only 3 or 4 times a week maximum without stressing your adrenal system. No? Do you get tired after a cup of java these days? Gee, your adrenals are falling apart and it's time to cut back. Thank God this only lasted 8 months of my life. I was sleep deprived, felt like a vampire but was doing better than anyone else I knew on such a schedule. Since I only had a 4 hour shift to work from 3:00 a.m. to 7:00 a.m. on weekends, I made up my lost 10 hours of sleep over weekends.

I always ate my 6 to 8 meals a day plus I worked out 2 or 3 times a week and got my rest. So no excuses. You have time. You just have to make it. The point is, it doesn't matter if you wake up at 4 o'clock in the afternoon because you work a midnight shift. Whatever time you arise, immediately begin eating 'breakfast' or whatever you want to call that first meal. Breakfast is the start of your day, the 'breaking of your fast' so to speak… So eat something! And continue to eat again at least every third hour you are awake, even if you are awake 36 hours in a row. Eat on time, no excuses. You can vary your feeding times, if necessary, catering to your work, sleep and exercise schedules, but anyone can at least make sure they are fitting in 6 meals and 6 hours of sleep each day (although 8 is best).

You know I am right. But it still sounds like too much trouble to you, eh? Look, if your primary excuse for failing to stick to this program is your laziness to pack a lunch or prepare and control your own food, or counting a few calories, and you insist that Met-rx or EAS powders are better for you than real food, then failure is your own fault. Don't EVER neglect to use the 12 Food Groups as a guide and NEVER under eat nor have less than 6 meals a day. TRUST ME ON THIS

ONE. You can sit around all day and blow off exercise.

But don't you dare tempt fate by shoveling tons of food down your neck NOR starving yourself believing that you won't get fat from it. Excess is excess and starving yourself shuts the metabolism down. And every day you put off exercise is another day that you will look in the mirror and complain about your fat gut, the cellulite, the bags under your eyes, your tummy pouch and everything else you secretly aren't too proud of. No, I am not psychic and I do not know you individually, so I am not personally assessing your condition. I do know how most people are though. I can't say how long it will take to correct what's wrong in anyone, but a day worked is a day gained, isn't it?

Do not write me and tell me this program failed you, I have made it as simple as anyone ever has right now. Only YOU can FAIL YOU on this or any other program. I, nor 'it', can fail you… The KNOW HOW is designed around how "Nature" works, not some marketing campaign and therefore I assure you, it cannot fail unless you refuse to accurately follow it! No amount of kicking, scratching, arguing or bogus propaganda is going to get your digestive system to work any better than I have explained it. I will say it until I die, if you aren't separating your foods, NO program will work for you! Well guess what? There is logic in everything you have tried before...

Low carb diets <u>are</u> only partially successful because they separate the carbs from the protein and fat sources (even though the diet eventually fails you because you DO need some carbs…Only not with your proteins and fats). If you are following the Atkins diet and have no muscle or have sagging skin, thank the good doctor who prescribed it… There's no saggy skin on this program.

Low fat diets work a little but it is only because they separate the fats from the carbs The failure of these plans stem from having your essential fats eliminated, eating too many carbohydrates and the fact you were still mixing proteins and carbs together. Have acne or menstrual issues? Still fat after months of effort? Have unbearable gas? Three strikes, you're out! If you mix your foods, you're going to end up protein malnourished. This only occurs when one, it isn't digesting or two, you're not eating as much protein as you should to begin with.

Most of the emails I get are from people telling me they already 'know how' to eat a 'healthy' diet and they 'look great' too, but in reality they are exaggerating or they wouldn't have contacted me to begin with. I look at their diets and it is amazing how many carbs people eat with their proteins. All the Zone Diet does in an attempt to remedy the high carb or fat deficient approach is cut your carbs in half by merely making it look as though you're doing something beneficial. Nothing more, nothing less, and it's obviously not enough. Like the vegetarians who have been mixing fats and carbs together forever, you become overweight or sickly looking despite lowering your calories.

It's not from a lack of protein, it's from mixing fats and carbs. I have had a lot of people tell me that they are on 40-30-30 Nutrition based program like the Zone that suggests eating chicken, rice and broccoli with a little olive oil too. I have just as many tell me that in the morning they have something like oatmeal with egg whites and maybe one yolk... You know the routine. Steak is a no-no for a low fat dieter though. Well, once either of them made the simple transition to having oatmeal and rice at separate feedings from the eggs and chicken, that's all it took for the magic to begin. I don't mean simply separately eating one bowl and heading to the other.

I mean eating 2 or 3 hours apart. Is it too much to ask for you to eat potatoes separate from steak if that means you're allowed steak again? But does the diet really work for everyone? Is it all things for all people? Yes it is. In fact, it even works for animals. Listen, do you have a pet? Well, I do. When we got him, he was 2 pounds. 2 years old and full grown. He's a half Chihuahua and half Jack Russell mix (don't ask, I don't know) but he was a little guy. 6 months later, he weighed nearly 6 pounds.

No, he didn't look malnourished when we got him, and no he doesn't look fat today. Since eating better, giving him vitamins, minerals, oils and good food, he is a completely different dog though. All we did was put him on our diet. Tequila (his name) eats proteins at one meal and grains at another. So does our other little one, Teaka, a teacup Chihuahua. She's 3 and a half pounds. The veterinarian told me that her breed doesn't normally exceed 2 pounds. What can I say? She eats right. Meats, vegetables, fruits, real food. So does my 3rd dog, Pookie. It amazes me how people can malnourish their dogs by feeding them 'dog' food and then wonder why the little guys are so full of ailments. But what's worse is that you do it to yourselves.

Unwittingly, we are malnourished, yet overfed and so unhealthy, but you don't even realize it. Another automobile analogy (can you tell I grew up next to a General Motors Plant?)… What is wrong with those people that go out of your way to put premium gas in their cars and regularly change its oil using, once again, only the best supplies? All that fuss but when it comes time to fueling up and cleaning out or adding the best ingredients nature has to offer to their own bodies, it's a different story. They still eat fast-processed, ready made, fat free foods and write off being fat, sick and unattractive on genetics. Proof is in the pudding. Speaking of pudding, I suppose if we expect them to actually get with the program we better give everyone some more ideas of what to eat!

Write down what you ate today because you're going to need this info in a minute:

Breakfast:

Brunch:

Lunch:

Mid-day:

Dinner:

Mid-Evening:

Other:

Supplements:

Notes:

HERE'S WHAT'S FOR BREAKFAST..

For breakfast, if you want carbohydrates (meaning you have decided upon having a low fat meal consisting of no meats or fats, only starches and fiber filled carbs), maybe you'll choose to have cereal, nonfat, NOT whole, 2% or 1%, but nonfat milk, and follow it up with a piece of fruit. You could even have a slice of toast with no sugar added jelly or nonstick pan fried hash browns with fat free butter on the side if you like (just do not fry the potatoes in oil or use real butter because carbohydrates can't be eaten with added fats). You could even have pancakes or waffles instead if you prefer, using pure maple syrup in small amounts, fresh berries and nonfat butter. Again, we don't use real butter with carb meals.

If you don't feel like carbohydrates, have a protein and fat meal like eggs and bacon with a side of diced mushrooms, onions, and peppers. The vegetables are essential and assist in digestion, eating just protein and fat alone will eventually backfire. In fact, you can treat yourself to a REAL OMELET using these guidelines. Take onions, peppers, mushrooms, broccoli and a piece of real cheese and place them in the fold of some eggs and you're all set! This then, is a perfect, animal source, protein and fat, therefore low carbohydrate meal. Remember, fibrous carbs are not the same as starchy carbs.

What about lunch? Have pasta if you want it! It's not evil. But because pasta is made of grains, it is a carbohydrate food, so instead of having it at dinner when carbohydrates are harder to digest for most people, have it earlier in the day, here at lunch when the body can more easily handle carbs. Make sure to not use any oil, butter or meat on it. You can still have all the garlic, spices and diced veggies you always do, but use nonfat sauce and nonfat Parmesan cheese instead.
On the side you could have garlic bread made with non-fat butter and fresh garlic, however, meatballs are to be eaten at anoth-

er meal all together. If you do decide to have meatballs, make sure they aren't made with bread crumbs (that's a starchy carb, a no-no with protein foods). In regards to nonfat butter, I do not mean margarine, I mean fat free butter. I assure you, non-fat butter exists. I get mine as a spray but there are other brands that come as spreads. Ask your grocer which they carry.

An alternative for lunch could be a bowl of rice, with black or red beans and steamed veggies on the side, topped by soy sauce. Do not add oil or meat to this dish either. It's a carbohydrate meal, so keep it low fat. You can however use nonfat broths to flavor the rice. Remember, 'non-animal based' meals of carbohydrates are to remain as low fat and vegetarian as possible in order to allow for proper digestion. You can only have carbohydrates with other carbohydrates. If you do not feel like carbohydrates for lunch, have some roasted chicken with a salad. You can use REAL cheese plus a little REAL dressing because low fat and nonfat dressings all contain sugars (which are carbs, and a no-no with meats). Also, you cannot have FRENCH FRIES with this meal either! Potatoes are carbohydrates and frying them in fat is a bad idea. Chicken and salad... That's a proper 'animal based' protein and fat meal!

TIP: I normally have salads when I go out to eat. Most people order their lunches from restaurants. This is important to note because a restaurant sometimes delivers extra food that exceeds your allowed calories and other times they add things that are off limit to your meal. Just because they do this doesn't mean you have to actually eat the extras. Keep your protein and fat meal low in carbohydrate. No fries, no croutons, no rice, no baked potatoes with meat...

You can have a potato with your rice or pasta meal anytime you like, you can even have it by itself, but you cannot use butter or cream (unless it is non-fat) and carbs are off limits to all protein meals. I order my potatoes 'dry' and take them home with me for a snack or something later. DINNER. You're always better off having fish, poultry or meat with steamed vegetables or another salad at this meal. Again, have your typical steak and potatoes dinner but without the potatoes! That means you're allowed more steak, so who loses with that sort of deal?

This plan goes for your kids too. Do not use the excuse that your kids want to eat different. KIDS EAT HOW YOU TELL THEM TO. Get used to eating this way then figure out on your own (you know them better than I do) how to get them on the program or they will be unhealthy and worried about their appearance when they grow up too. If you allow that to happen, you're an awful human being. I truly feel that way. My child's health means the world to me. Not having control over what your kids eat, like in the case of separate households, is one thing. But if you have any say so whatsoever, enforce it. You know what is right or wrong. Forget about the high self-esteem that comes from looking trim and fit… Without good health we have nothing.

What we have done to this point is cover your three main meals. Breakfast, lunch and dinner. Next, let's discuss your snacks. Plan on eating one between breakfast and lunch then another between lunch and dinner and one more between dinner and bedtime. Keep one rule in mind when selecting a snack..

You can't have two carbohydrate feedings in a row.

Having two carb meals in a row triggers a negative chain reaction inside of you that tells the body to burn muscle tissue and store fat, which is obviously undesirable. Interestingly enough, having two protein and fat meals in a row, is optimal, because it gets your body burning fat and building muscle. For this reason, I schedule one carbohydrate meal in the AM (either breakfast or brunch) and the other lunch or mid-day, depending on when the first one was eaten. So, for snacks, if your breakfast was full of carbohydrates, you should have protein snacks of cottage cheese, or almond butter (no sugar added) mixed with whey protein and Lemmon's Oil on celery at brunch. If breakfast was protein and fat based, then a snack of bagels and fruit would work. But if you have carbs mid morning, you can't have them at lunch. In my opinion, breakfast and lunch are the best times to have carbs.

Mid-day, if lunch was a carbohydrate meal, you could have coffee with heavy cream, pure whey protein and spinach or broccoli to follow down the hatch too. It's a good habit to always have greens in the freezer at home or work if need be. Sure, it sounds crazy to eat greens at every meal, but it works wonders on healing your gut and clearing the intestines. If I had protein at lunch, like a salad I ordered from a restaurant, this is when I will eat my baked potato that came with it. I sometimes get an extra potato or bring a bowl of beans for these 'meals between meals'.

Mid-evening. I cannot insist upon you're eating a mid-evening snack often enough. Mine is usually scrambled eggs, but I always have a protein meal as a final feeding. It speeds the metabolism like you'll never know unless you try it for a few weeks.

TIP: Never have more than one whey drink a day and never use a meal replacement powder or protein bar. The body was designed to run off food, not cookie dough and cake batter... If you only use what I recommend then you cannot fail. If you eat any other supplements, I cannot assure you of anything.

All those high protein, low carb bars are junk food too. If it tastes like candy, it is candy. If it isn't, then prove it to me. Don't send me sales literature as though that's some sort of proof, it isn't. Send me actual proof. You can't. And like it or not, there isn't a single bar that's as good for you as real food and since most 'health food' bars are made by candy companies anyhow, you really haven't a clue as to what's in them (glycerine IS a carb). At best, your 'meal replacements' are nothing more than expensive after-workout snacks. It is 100% absolutely true that you can become firm WITHOUT magic potions, protein powders and caffeine tablets.... Forget what the ads say! Throw it all away! Get a refund! Why would the 'establishment' and supplement salesmen want to hide things from you? Because if you knew the truth it would put an end to a billion dollar business.

You wouldn't visit a fat farm clinic or QUACK doctors that peddle things like Phen Phen if you knew the truth so these companies suppress the info that would otherwise deter you from their services. It would also put many pharmaceutical companies out of the picture. In their defense, most companies haven't even a clue what they are doing to begin with. It's just big business to them. That doesn't make it better, but it does explain a lot. Dishonest people are driven by the all mighty dollar and many of the folks out marketing the hottest fat loss products available only know about, you guessed it, making money. Not nutrition. Not exercise. They have made their livings their entire lives telling people what they want to hear to sell anything from floor cleaners, car wax and protein powders.

THREE MONTHS OF MENUS

REMINDER: Breakfast is best eaten immediately upon waking. Lunch can be eaten at what you determine is your regular time. Dinner too can be eaten at your regular time. However, this is important, Brunch has to be eaten half way between Breakfast and Lunch. If you eat at 7:00 a.m. and 12:30 p.m. then Brunch should be scheduled in the middle at 9:45 a.m. Your Mid Day Snack is then also eaten half way between two meals, Lunch and Dinner. If you eat at 12:30 p.m. and 6:00 p.m. then schedule this snack at 3:15 p.m. right in the middle. Your Mid Evening Snack is then to be sandwiched half way between Dinner and bedtime on non-workout days. Say you're normally having dinner at 6:00 p.m. and hitting the hay at 11:00 p.m. then you must eat a snack at 8:30 p.m. nightly.

Using this guide, go ahead and follow each menu for a week. Take the time you have now to figure out what kinks that are in your current schedule so you 'set' regular daily eating times. Each menu technically also includes an 'After Workout' snack for having on your workout days. I personally like to have a little more food those days.

My pre-workout meal is usually nothing more than whey protein, coffee and cream. It may be steak and spinach. If I am in a rush, like first thing in the morning, it's definitely whey and cream because I need it fast and I would never workout on an empty belly. I will also save the carbs for after the session and typically only have half of what's considered a normal sized meal. My regular feedings are 600 calories or so. My 'after workout' meals are only 300. Keep your own caloric requirements in mind while figuring up these diets for the weeks to come.

DON LEMMON'S MENU NUMBER ONE!

Breakfast:
Eggs, Bacon, Mushrooms, Onions and Cottage Cheese.
2 Don Lemmon Multi Nutrient Support Capsules.

Brunch:
Oats, Raw Unsweetened Cocoa and Maple Syrup.

Lunch:
Steak, Spinach, Peppers, Chicken Broth, Herbal Tea, Cream.
2 Don Lemmon Multi Nutrient Support Capsules.

Mid-Day Snack:
Tomato, Basil and Onion Bread with Rice and Black Beans.

Dinner:
Chicken, Spinach, Bleu Cheese, Lemmon's Oil.
2 Don Lemmon Multi Nutrient Support Capsules.

After Workout:
Bagel with Nonfat Cream Cheese.

Mid-Evening Snack:
Tuna, Tea, Heavy Cream, and Celery w/Pumpkin Butter.

NOTES:

DON LEMMON'S MENU NUMBER TWO!

Breakfast:
Grits, Banana, and Nonfat Milk.
2 Don Lemmon Multi Nutrient Support Capsules.

Brunch:
Tuna, Cheddar Cheese, Diced Olives, Cabbage.

Lunch:
Chicken, Bok Choy, Olive Oil, and Garlic.
2 Don Lemmon Multi Nutrient Support Capsules.

Mid-Day Snack:
Rice, Salsa, and Red Beans.

Dinner:
Steak, Sugar Free BBQ Sauce, Broccoli, Lemmon's Oil.
2 Don Lemmon Multi Nutrient Support Capsules.

After Workout:
English Muffin, Tufo Turkey Slice, and Nonfat Cheese.

Mid-Evening Snack:
Deviled Eggs - Mustard, Sour Cream, Vinegar, Paprika, Olives, Pimentos, Lemmon's Oil, Yolks, Boiled Egg Whites.

NOTES: _____

_____

_____

_____

_____

_____

_____

DON LEMMON'S MENU NUMBER THREE!

Breakfast:
Whole Wheat Toast, Blueberry Jelly, Hash Browns, and Apple.
2 Don Lemmon Multi Nutrient Support Capsules.

Brunch:
Omelet - Eggs, Cheese, diced Ham, Onions and Peppers.

Lunch:
Rice, Soy Sauce, and Snow Peas.
2 Don Lemmon Multi Nutrient Support Capsules.

Mid-Day Snack:
Cottage Cheese, Lemmon's Oil, Ginger and Cinnamon.

Dinner:
Scallops, Brussel Sprouts, Herbs and Butter.
2 Don Lemmon Multi Nutrient Support Capsules.

After Workout:
Lima Beans and Corn.

Mid-Evening Snack:
Extra Firm Tofu, Lemmon's Oil and Green Beans.

NOTES:

DON LEMMON'S MENU NUMBER FOUR!

Breakfast:
Scrambled Eggs, Broccoli, Herbal Tea.
2 Don Lemmon Multi Nutrient Support Capsules.

Brunch:
Natural Peanut Butter Puffed Cereal and NonFat Milk.

Lunch:
Ground Beef, Collard Greens and Lemmon's Oil.
2 Don Lemmon Multi Nutrient Support Capsules.

Mid-day Snack:
Whey Protein, Vanilla Flavor and low carb Soy Drink.

Dinner:
Tuna, Mayo, Relish, Olives, Celery, Mozzarella, Romaine Lettuce. 2
Don Lemmon Multi Nutrient Support Capsules.

After Workout:
98% Fat Free Vegetarian Pizza.

Mid-Evening Snack:
Shrimp, Un-Sweetened Sauce, melted Coconut Butter.

NOTES: _____

_____

_____

_____

_____

_____

_____

DON LEMMON'S MENU NUMBER FIVE!

Breakfast:
Natural Decaf Coffee, Toasted Oats, Nonfat Milk, and Prunes.
2 Don Lemmon Multi Nutrient Support Capsules.

Brunch:
Hard-boiled Eggs, Sea Salt, Pepper, and Raw Broccoli.

Lunch:
Cornbread, Strawberries, and Pinto Beans.
2 Don Lemmon Multi Nutrient Support Capsules.

Mid-Day Snack:
Turkey, Mustard Greens, Lemmon's Oil.

Dinner:
Chicken, Asparagus, Garlic, Lemmon's Oil.
2 Don Lemmon Multi Nutrient Support Capsules.

After Workout:
Peaches, Unsweetened Jello, and a Fiber Supplement.

Mid-Evening Snack:
Ham and grilled mixed Peppers.

NOTES:

DON LEMMON'S MENU NUMBER SIX!

Breakfast:
Creamed Wheat, All Spice, Raisins, Apple and Nonfat Milk.
2 Don Lemmon Multi Nutrient Support Capsules.

Brunch:
Naturally Decaf Coffee high speed blended with Whey Protein.

Lunch:
Peas, Kidney Beans, Yam, and Italian Bread.
2 Don Lemmon Multi Nutrient Support Capsules.

Mid-Day Snack:
Cashew Butter, Pumpkin Butter, mixed with Whey Protein.

Dinner:
Steak, diced Bacon, Lemmon's Oil, and fresh Wax Beans.
2 Don Lemmon Multi Nutrient Support Capsules.

After Workout:
Sliced baked Potatoes, and Salsa to dip it in.

Mid-Evening Snack:
Smoked Salmon, diced fried Celery and Onions.

NOTES: _____

_____

_____

_____

_____

_____

_____

DON LEMMON'S MENU NUMBER SIX!

Breakfast:
Creamed Wheat, All Spice, Raisins, Apple and Nonfat Milk.
2 Don Lemmon Multi Nutrient Support Capsules.

Brunch:
Naturally Decaf Coffee high speed blended with Whey Protein.

Lunch:
Peas, Kidney Beans, Yam, and Italian Bread.
2 Don Lemmon Multi Nutrient Support Capsules.

Mid-Day Snack:
Cashew Butter, Pumpkin Butter, mixed with Whey Protein.

Dinner:
Steak, diced Bacon, Lemmon's Oil, and fresh Wax Beans.
2 Don Lemmon Multi Nutrient Support Capsules.

After Workout:
Sliced baked Potatoes, and Salsa to dip it in.

Mid-Evening Snack:
Smoked Salmon, diced fried Celery and Onions.

NOTES: _____

_____

_____

_____

_____

_____

_____

DON LEMMON'S MENU NUMBER SEVEN!

Breakfast:
Eggs Over Easy, Turkey Sausage, and regular Tea.
2 Don Lemmon Multi Nutrient Support Capsules.

Brunch:
Almond Butter w/ Lemmon's Oil, Whey Protein, on Celery.

Lunch:
Wild Rice, steamed Cauliflower, and Kidney Beans.
2 Don Lemmon Multi Nutrient Support Capsules.

Mid-Day Snack:
No Sugar Beef Jerky, raw Chinese Broccoli

Dinner:
Cat Fish, Parmesan Cheese, Green Leafy Salad, and Radishes.
2 Don Lemmon Multi Nutrient Support Capsules.

After Workout:
Nonfat Vanilla Yogurt and baked Sweet Potato.

Mid-Evening Snack:
Chicken Wings, Raw Broccoli, and Bleu Cheese Dressing.

NOTES: _____

_____

_____

_____

_____

_____

_____

DON LEMMON'S MENU NUMBER EIGHT!

Breakfast:
Corn Grits, Oat Bran toast, no sugar added Elder Berry jelly.
2 Don Lemmon Multi Nutrient Support Capsules.

Brunch:
Cottage Cheese, Lemmon's Oil and Natural Decaf Coffee.

Lunch:
Steak Strips on a bed of Romaine Lettuce and Cheddar Cheese.
2 Don Lemmon Multi Nutrient Support Capsules.

Mid-Day Snack:
Diced Banana, Pear, Cantaloupe, and nonfat Cookie.

Dinner:
Baked Salmon, Rosemary, Dijon Mustard, and Red Lettuce.
2 Don Lemmon Multi Nutrient Support Capsules.

After Workout:
Fat Free Cheddar Crackers and a glass of Grape juice.

Mid-Evening Snack:
Herb Tea, Whey Protein, and Heavy Cream.

NOTES:

DON LEMMON'S MENU NUMBER NINE!

Breakfast:
Natural Cocoa cereal, Nonfat milk, and Peach.
2 Don Lemmon Multi Nutrient Support Capsules.

Brunch:
Soy Sausages, grilled Onion, and Butter.

Lunch:
Nonfat Grilled Cheese Sandwich and Tomato Soup.
2 Don Lemmon Multi Nutrient Support Capsules.

Mid-Day Snack:
Chicken Breasts, Lemmon's Oil, unsweetened Cole Slaw.

Dinner:
Baked Potatoes, Vanilla Yogurt, Soy Bits, and Mushrooms.
2 Don Lemmon Multi Nutrient Support Capsules.

After Workout:
Crumpets, Raspberries, Nonfat Yogurt.

Mid-Evening Meal:
Pickled Eggs and Lemmon's Oil.

NOTES:

DON LEMMON'S MENU NUMBER TEN!

Breakfast:
Pancakes, Maple Syrup, and diced Mangoes.
2 Don Lemmon Multi Nutrient Support Capsules.

Brunch:
Roast Beef and Provolone slices.

Lunch:
Egg-less Noodles, Nonfat Cream of Mushroom Soup, Spinach.
2 Don Lemmon Multi Nutrient Support Capsules.

Mid-Day Snack:
Whey Protein, Banana Crème flavored Coffee with Cream.

Dinner:
Grilled Liver and Caesar salad.
2 Don Lemmon Multi Nutrient Support Capsules.

After Workout:
3 different colored Rices, Beans and Squashes mixed.

Mid-Evening Snack:
Eggs folded over cheddar cheese, Coconut Butter, and salsa.

NOTES:

DON LEMMON'S MENU NUMBER ELEVEN!

Breakfast:
Poached Eggs, Cheese Sauce, Tea, fried Onions and Peppers.
2 Don Lemmon Multi Nutrient Support Capsules.

Brunch:
Nonfat Milk, Toast and Low Fat Peanut spread.

Lunch:
Diced Ham, Mayo, Lemmon's Oil on Romaine Lettuce.
2 Don Lemmon Multi Nutrient Support Capsules.

Mid-Day Snack:
Meatless Vegetable Stew.

Dinner:
Scallops, Almonds, Butter, and Broccoli.
2 Don Lemmon Multi Nutrient Support Capsules.

After Workout:
Non-fat Swiss Cheese on Rye with a Soy Ham slice and Beets.

Mid-Evening Snack:
Baked Chicken Legs, boiled Spinach, Lemmon's Oil, Garlic.

NOTES: _____

_____

_____

_____

_____

_____

_____

DON LEMMON'S MENU NUMBER TWELVE!

Breakfast:
Eggs, Jack Cheese, Mushroom, Turmeric, and Sea Salt.
2 Don Lemmon Multi Nutrient Support Capsules.

Brunch:
Cherries, Strawberries, Kiwis, and Orange slices w/ Mint.

Lunch:
Chicken Thighs, Portabella Mushrooms, Basil and Oregano.
2 Don Lemmon Multi Nutrient Support Capsules.

Mid-Day Snack:
Spiral Pasta with Fat Free Italian Dressing and Broccoli.

Dinner:
Trout, Shallots, Cloves, Peppers, Parsley and Lemmon's Oil.
2 Don Lemmon Multi Nutrient Support Capsules.

After Workout:
Green apple baked with all spice and raw brown cane sugar.

Mid-Evening Snack:
Pine Nuts and Extra Firm Tofu with Soy Sauce.

NOTES: _____

_____

_____

_____

_____

_____

_____

DON LEMMON'S MENU NUMBER THIRTEEN!

Breakfast:
Oatmeal, Nonfat Milk, frozen Blue Berries.
2 Don Lemmon Multi Nutrient Support Capsules.

Brunch:
Cottage Cheese, Lemmon's Oil and All Spice.

Lunch:
Broiled Steak and Spinach Caesar Salad.
2 Don Lemmon Multi Nutrient Support Capsules.

Mid-Day Snack:
Pure White Rice and boiled Seaweed.

Dinner:
Roasted Chicken, Olive Oil, mixed Italian Vegetables.
2 Don Lemmon Multi Nutrient Support Capsules.

After Workout:
Vegetarian Macaroni and Cheese.

Mid-Evening Snack:
Scrambled Eggs mixed with diced veggies and Cream.

NOTES: _____

_____

_____

_____

_____

_____

_____

A LITTLE COOKING ADVICE

The 12 Food Groups give you plenty of different items to select from but the foods listed aren't the only ones you are allowed to eat. No way. There are a wide variety of other foods to choose from that fall into those same categories. You can use almost any one of them to devise your own diet and wean out of old eating habits, just compare notes. If you make sure you've paid attention to what the appropriate food categories are at all times by using the 12 Food Groups as a lifestyle guide, you cannot fail. A goose and a squirrel may not be the same things as a steak or a chicken, but they are certainly the same type of foods. They are protein and fat sources.

Nuts and seeds aren't the same, but they are close. If you don't like nuts, have seeds instead. Just review the food groups when necessary and you'll be fine. In fact, email and ask me anytime if you get confused. By following these diets over the next 13 weeks you will not only get yourself into shape but you will possibly discover tastes for different foods you didn't know you had. However, you may not be so open to new things and want to change a particular item here and there.

That's fine. These menus are interchangeable. If you do not like a particular food, then go to the 12 Food Groups and select another one from that particular 'group' to replace it with. If there is a carb you don't like, replace it with another carb. Exchange protein for protein, fat for fat, etc. etc. Even if you want to have a different protein meal one week that you saw on another one of the menus, simply switch it with the protein meal on your current one, or carb for carb, etc. and so on. Sometimes, certain foods may even seem a bit expensive, depending on the season, and other times, you'll change a meal because you're eating on the run. I understand.

Just stick with the 'like' for 'like' idea. Replace carbs for carbs, proteins and fats for protein and fats. As far as expense goes, I used to get canned tuna instead of fresh tuna and sometimes we got green beans instead of broccoli. For the most part though, you will discover that foods bought at a store are much more affordable than the ones at restaurants. Fish is fish, red meat is red meat, beans are beans, fruits are fruits, but not if you buy them at a gas station or restaurant instead of a grocery store. Stick with the most natural sources of food you can afford, whenever you shop and all will be fine.

How practical is this plan? When we go grocery shopping, we grab a couple containers of oatmeal, a gallon of nonfat milk and a few bags of frozen berries for breakfast. That is about $12 for a week's worth. We also get seven 32 ounce containers of nonfat cottage cheese to mix with one and one half tablespoons of Lemmon's Oil. At $2.50 a container and a third bottle of oil (10 servings) for $4, that's another $20. A bag of rice and a bag of beans, plus a little bouillon and soy sauce is $5 at the most total for the week. We have cream in our herbal tea during the afternoon with a can of tuna and that's about $5 a week for the fish and $3 for cream.

Next we get some chicken, steak or salmon, a pound a day at no more than $2.99 a pound, a little container of feta cheese, lettuce and mix it at home with one and a half tablespoons of Lemmon's Oil for dinner. That's $30 a week maximum. Eggs and broccoli are the last meal so we grab seven bags of 99 cent veggies and seven 18-packs of eggs for $1.50 each. That's $18 for the week. I suppose since we use 2 bottles of multi-nutrients a month too we can call that another $10 a week between us. Add it up. That's basically $60 a week for an athletic man for both food and supplements. $200 a month for food, $50 for supplements. See, it's extremely practical.

So, start today with whichever menu you want, even if you configure one of your own based upon likes, dislikes, budget or convenience. Do not forget, each meal is to be equal in calories.

Only you know how many calories a day are required if you've done the math earlier in the book. Divide those calories by six and that's your per-meal allowance. You did do that didn't you? I wrote this book for you because I wanted you to use it to succeed. But all I can do is explain things to you using the best methods I know.

I still cannot twist your arm to do the foot work. Besides, if I get hit by a bus, this book and the prescribed homework is all you'll have to remember me by. So depend upon yourself. Not me or anyone else. I cannot guarantee your success unless you can guarantee that you will take appropriate action. I do not know what you are going to do with what I gave you, but one thing is for sure, do not expect anyone else to make the changes we've discussed for you. This is YOUR gig and YOUR gig alone.

Anytime you need a reminder or an added bit of motivation, feel free to write me, but read and reread this book as often as necessary to commit it to habit. You know what's in it for you if you do. You'll become healthier and successful. I didn't settle for less than that myself when I started so now it's your turn to get on the ball. You have already set a goal for yourself and now it's high time you began working to attain it. How long will it take to reach your goals once you start? That depends on your current condition. You could gain 20 pounds of muscle in 40 days if you need it or you could lose 100 pounds of fat in 6 months if that's what is necessary.

All things take time, but fortunately for you, not as much time as it would using other methods. Just remember, no added sugars (like in juices and canned products) or processed oils (like in peanut butters and processed cheeses) or fake sugars (in gum and fat free products) or any of these un-natural additives in anything you buy from now on. No, this doesn't limit your ability to eat flavored foods.

You will discover that even by adding just a couple of spices to a meal, you can experiment with virtually anything to flavor your meals. I sparingly use sea salt (which contains dozens of minerals and will not cause water retention) and ground black pepper on almost everything I eat. I love garlic too and I eat a lot of that, but it's a preference to smell so Greek! I also like 'hot' stuff like spicy mustard (wasabi) and chili sauce. We love our spicy cheese dips, soy sauce, low sodium broths, unsweetened catsup, yellow mustard, and steak spices are all great to keep on hand. If you aren't familiar with some of the spices I have listed, that's alright. Your grocer should be. Ask a clerk at your store where to find them.

As far as cooking utensils to prepare your foods, most adults should know how to cook (although I am never surprised these days at how many people do not know the simplest of things). I get by using plastic measuring cups, spoons, knives, forks, plastic containers, bowls, plates, a microwave, blender, frying pan, spatula, boiling pot, strainer and a big stirring spoon. Some of you might want more than this. If so, pick up any other items you may find listed in a recipe book or that you learn of somewhere else the next time you're out shopping! I have a peanut butter maker and rice cooker myself. That's about as exotic as I get. If you are still one of those people who say there is no time to cook, mass prepare your food twice a week. There, no more excuses.

Some things like oatmeal or scrambled eggs I cook the same day, but I might crack my eggs the night before or dice my veggies twice a week. I will grill chicken and steak once a week but make my broccoli daily. I refrigerate or freeze whatever I cook that that won't be used for a few days then simply pull it out and microwave it when I want to eat. Another example, we make soup out of virtually anything we can buy from the produce section of the grocery store. We use beets w/tops, carrots w/tops, garlic, celery, parsley, garlic, okra, squash, garlic, water, more garlic, onions, meat... boil, add garlic and then we eat!

It's a soup that not only tastes good, but cleans our systems out as well. It's easy to make and if frozen, lasts as long as we need it. So get off your but and cook some food! Preparing your own meals can be both easy and fun plus awfully tasty if you pay close attention to the ingredients you choose. Using sensible flavorings on even foods that you normally wouldn't go near could end up making them some of your new favorite dishes.

Beware, it is possible to add too much of a seemingly innocent ingredient and destroy the taste of an entire meal. if you dump too much salt on a pasta dish or if you add oregano to your oatmeal or by adding sugar to protein. This is most likely because far too many companies out there slip bleached sugars into our foods and spices. You better begin reading EVERY THING before placing it on your food or in your mouth. You CAN learn from your mistakes. Become aware of your every move. So if you add sugar to a protein by accident, that doesn't make it acceptable to eat. You can't digest a protein with sugar on it efficiently.

For example, one morning, I added cinnamon to my whole fat cottage cheese and the particular brand of cinnamon I used had sugar in it. I ended up throwing it all out. I also refuse to put sugar on anything including my cereal and coffee. Sugar literally disrupts your digestive system. Just about every spice you find at the store can be used with the exception of products with added sugar. Look at what you have now in the cupboard to see if all your choices truly are sugar free (artificial sweeteners are off limits as well).

If you feel the need to use any sugar at all for a recipe, you should only use the purest sources possible, like real honey, maple syrup or unbleached raw cane sugars... Even that white fructose which is sold in 'health' food stores is bad. So do your best to cut back in all areas of added sweeteners.

Sugars tend to cause ALL other foods containing them to ferment in your gut and remain undigested. That leads to all sorts of other degenerative disorders. Reversible disorders, yes, but that's no reason to subject yourself to the torture to begin with. Your best bet is to avoid all sweet and "white" colored food products to begin with so there is nothing left to question. If you want to use sugar just because you think the taste of real food is boring, GROW UP.

Get used to eating without additives for a change. Use little spicy twists and you can make any 'bland' old food taste more "socially appealing." If you're only excuse for cheating is because of taste, spices are one of the safest and most cost effective preventive measures against cheating. Refusing to eat 'right' because things aren't 'sweet' enough is sure evidence of your chemical addictions to food. Try cooking at home on your own today and you'll see! Just watch what you put in your mouth. Common sense dictates that if bacteria won't digest a cup cake then what makes you think your stomach will? Who can deny the exciting fringe benefits here?

You get to continue to eat whatever it is that you already do eat, but somehow, this program magically allows you to succeed for a change by merely separating your foods into appropriate meal patterns. How could ANYONE have a problem with that? You're going to eat what you want to anyhow! At least with me, you're allowed! You would have to be insane to not give it a try! The same foods you like to eat now, only at different meals.

Some flavorings will change calorie intakes. With that said, don't forget to count your calories, watch your grams of fat, carbohydrates, and proteins closely, and read the labels of everything you put in your mouth from now on. Most food labels list serving size (measure), servings per container (how many), calories per serving (you may be having more or less than one serving so read this), total fat (per serving), total carbohydrates (per serving), and total protein (per serving). Also read the actual ingredient list. Hydrogenated anything or syrups or sugars or stuff ending in 'ose' is a no-no. Only YOU can watch out for YOU.

I want you to succeed. But I can only show you how. I cannot force you to do what I recommend. I hope you do not expect anyone else to make the changes for you. YOU make change and the people around you will make change. I know some of you have been blaming everything and everyone around you rather than looking to yourself for the source of the problem. Try taking some initiative. Stick out your chest. Hold up your head up and be willing to get your hands dirty. If that is too much for you right now, give this book to someone who is ready to put their past behind them and restructure their future. I WAS LIKE THIS TOO at one time! You're not alone!

FEELING BLOATED HAPPENS

What then should you expect to experience once you begin? Well, at first, you might experience some discomfort. I know, that's not a good feeling. You'll think the devil got a hold of you and that Don Lemmon is the patron demon, but stick it out anyhow. Your metabolism is slow right now. It takes a few days, maybe even a week or two for your body to regulate its sluggish behavior. This has nothing to do with salt. Sodium isn't related to holding water unless you haven't been using it for a prolonged period.

Sooner than later the bloating will disappear on it's own but only if you stick it out. Just divide your age by 3 and that is about how many days it should take for your body to adjust to eating properly. By then you will not only 'know' the program is working, you'll 'feel' it and SEE IT. Either way, keep in mind the bloating is all fairly typical. You WILL drop body fat during this 'grace' period, despite the fact you're 'feeling' otherwise. What causes it? The bloating is caused for the most part by your backed up bowels.

No worries, just relax, within a week, that will change. You will start noticing positive changes in your regularity and feel fine once the metabolism speeds back up. Whatever you do, DO NOT QUIT due to this bloating! If you quit, every single time you try to start the program over again, you will bloat ALL OVER AGAIN! The bloating is a false feeling that the program isn't working. Just ride it out for the time being and no matter how nasty, oily, gross and fat you feel, ignore it. This is the body's only means by which it knows to dump toxins and shift into metabolic over-drive. It's like taking your car up a steep hill.

It's tough going up, but once you're at the top, it's always a breeze coming down! Besides, you can literally vary your grocery list any way you like from now on. You picked the foods.

You can even increase the variety in your diet using the rules we have learned so far. If all you're doing is eating what you always have, but you haven't seen any change until now… Things inside of you are FINALLY changing… So don't blow it by quitting. I don't care if you're bloated all month. Stick it out. I simply ask you watch what you eat and that you refuse to have junk food any longer. Not a single physician on Earth is going to say that's asking too much. In fact, talk to one.

Your physician will agree with everything written so far... Eating clean, exercising regularly, drinking fresh water, sleeping longer, only taking supplements that include vitamins, minerals and essential fatty acids and sticking with it the rest of your life... What's not to agree with? If your doctor says my diet sounds like bull, ask him to see his abdominal muscles. Are they visible? What kind of shape is your 'doctor' in? Can he out run most people his age? Out weight lift them? I think you can tell if their advice is worth taking or not regarding this matter.

If they tell you that it's normal to crave hydrogenated oils and artificial sweeteners, that chlorine in your water is fine, a lack of sleep and exercise is acceptable, or that junk food is 'OK' by them too, it is time to switch doctors! I cannot begin to tell you how many elderly people have seen their cholesterol come under control or how many teenagers saw their pimples disappear by simply dropping the junk food and following the instructions in the next chapter to get those poisons out of you even faster. I have plead my case. Now get started. In case you do not think that constipation or bloating has anything to do with making progress... Or your grandparent's cholesterol problems…

HOW CHOLESTEROL REALLY RAISES

I hope those of you who think constipation has nothing to do with many of your body's ailments and are living miserable, limited and inactive lives are only going to get worse in elderly life, if you make it that long. You will more likely die an early death. If you didn't look as bad as you do now 20 years ago, what will you look like in another 20 years? Young and old, male and female alike, hear me now… If you do not have large, full and 'healthy' bowel movements regularly (twice a day…), then ask yourself, "Am I sure I am eating ENOUGH food?" Because no matter what you believe causes constipation or, like far too many people believe, that it will go away on it's own eventually, step one is eating more food.

If you want to feel better than you do now and know you need cleaned out on a more regular basis, all you have to do is make certain you are eating enough food for the most part. I assume you're already going to separate your foods correctly, but skipping meals, not eating your vegetables and cutting the calories back doesn't help you in the bathroom. That is unless of course you want stinky, milky, pasty, blotchy, dry, purple-ish looking, and easily bruising skin. Do you have high blood pressure, oily flesh, mid-day headaches or plan your day around potential bowel movements that never happen? These are all sure signs that you're still 'backed' up even if you do 'go' every day.

Ever wonder why some people you know look like they have aged 20 years in under a decade? Sure, they may be smokers or drinkers or what not, but grandpa didn't go from hearty and healthy in stature to bony with a bloated abdomen for any other reason. He is literally full of crap from his years of constipation. Even if you are young, even if you have nice abs, if you have a bloated gut like a gorilla, you too are full of intestine clogging feces.

Your health is going to get really bad because your immune system can't fight the toxins in your bowel fast enough to defend the rest of the body in this condition. You lose muscle and your belly only gets bigger and bigger as the colon loses more and more control. I spent a lot of time on the crapper straining my brains out from as early as I could remember to as late in life as being on this diet full time. I would get gas so bad as a kid my parents would sit me on the toilet and wouldn't let me leave until there was evidence in the bowl that my bowel was empty. I was there so long at times my legs would fall asleep. I continued struggling with my movements until I was 21 or 22.

I know, that's not something any of us want to admit, but if I can do it, I think you can come forth too. It's time we do something to remedy the issue. Let me tell you something else, it's not what comes out, but what is left behind that hurts you. What goes in must come out. Think about 'that' for a moment. If the body was supposed to store it's 'waste' inside of you, there wouldn't be a process to drop it out your backside to begin with, and it would-n't be so uncomfortable for you when it doesn't. No, it's not 'nor-mal' to struggle to have a bowel movement.

If constipation, diarrhea or the feeling you're giving birth every time you want to go poo-poo has been plaguing you, it may be time to give mother nature a hand. No? Well, what you're doing now isn't working is it? Listen to your body. It's giving you a subliminal mes-sage. "Clean me… Clean me…" Seriously. The colon needs to be cleaned inside and out. Just to make sure we erase the errors of your past, I suggest you begin by performing a regular series of daily ene-mas for a short period of time. Don't kid yourself.

If you are constipated, you are toxic, and the fastest route to detoxifying the body after straightening the diet up is by giving yourself a good pipe cleaning. Sorry, fiber supplements aren't enough to solve your problem. Fiber helps to prevent further constipation, but if all you needed is 'more' fiber right now, we wouldn't be here. Why doesn't it? Because fiber doesn't dislodge what's trapped in there. It merely gets the fresh stuff past the crusty parts. The solution? Go out to the local drug store today and buy a half-gallon enema bag. It looks like a hot water bottle. Ask your pharmacist where in the store you can find one and do not be embarrassed by it.

Later the same day, when you're all alone and have your nerve worked up, fill the bag with 7 cups warm water, 1 cup freshly brewed coffee and hang it from a towel or coat rack near the toilet. Yes, that is 56 ounces of water and 8 ounces of coffee. Keep saying to yourself, "It's a bath for inside my butt." The caffeine goes in and 'challenges' -as they say- the liver to release it's backed up funk and bile. Bile is useful in many ways, but it's not meant to be backed up. Bile is supposed to emulsify the fats in our foods and is also a means by which toxins are eliminated from the body. Sometimes it just can't do it and usually it is because you're backed up. Are you burping, belching or bloated after you eat fats?

This is not only a sign that bile is backed up but now its led to having gall bladder problems. Not good. This can become quite serious, especially if you live in a polluted community. If you work or live in a polluted environment (which can be anywhere these days), things are absorbed into the lungs when you breath and then get dumped into the liver. This organ is sort of like the oil filter in your car and it wasn't meant to be abused. Things get worse when your community uses a lot of chlorine and fluoride in its water supply.

After you eat, drink and breath the body is supposed to efficiently pull toxins out of your blood and mix them with bile to be carried out through the 'regular' digestive process. Sometimes bile gets backed up because the metabolism has become sluggish. This is why your skin looks so awful, your breath is so bad, and most everything else including your joints may be ailing you. You're toxic and enemas are the easiest way to get your system going again. You see, bile is composed of salts, cholesterol and lecithin (the latter two are essential fats). When hydrogenated oils, which are bad sources of dietary cholesterol are eaten, they throw a monkey wrench into your bile's mix.

Usually good cholesterol is turned into a bile 'salt' which thins the mix. Hydrogenated oils are found in non-dairy creamers, lards, margarine and creamy peanut butters. When these fake fats are produced, it is done so by destroying natural foods, chemically converting them to longer lasting substances the body was never designed to digest. In fact, most countries in Europe BAN these things because they are so harmful to us. Some bile salts are secreted into the small intestine and eventually reabsorbed after circulation by the liver again. This could be good or bad because the enzyme 7-cholesterol dehydrogenase is regulated by the amount of salts returning through this process.

The more 'bad' salts that are made from 'bad' fats and the more that are secreted, the more that are reabsorbed, the slower the production of 'clean' salts from 'good' cholesterol becomes, and the higher your bad cholesterol levels increase. All because you're backed up and there is no 'exit' route for the waste to excrete itself properly. The conversion, circulation, production and excretion process of bile, toxins, cholesterol and waste depends upon eating, sleeping, fluids, anti-oxidants, b-complex vitamins, essential fatty acids… AND….

Taurine (taurocholic acid), glycine (glycocholic acid), copper (which are all found in large enough quantities in the Don Lemmon Multi-Nutrient for this reason). The final point there is that the efficiency of the body's ability to keep itself clean is not only based upon your regularity, but what you do to enforce it and what nutrients you are missing. This is why sometimes you get diarrhea and sometimes the bowels look green. The green is the bile finally dumping itself out and the diarrhea is the body liquefying your bowels to squeeze what waste it can out through your clogged pipes.

It's disgusting to think about and it's irritating to remember the last time it's happened, I know. But this is only happening because we aren't taught anything about proper bowel movements growing up, in school or by our physicians. It is a forgotten part of the health care system and it's why our children are having their appendix removed so early in life (or at all). The body knows it must keep itself clean even if you try to keep it backed up all the time. But it's not 'normal.' For now, if it happens, let the diarrhea pass and allow the body to eliminate itself the best it knows how. Take NOTHING to stop it. You have to let yourself clear out 'naturally' this one last time.

Now is not a time for fiber. Again, fiber allows you to go easier NEXT TIME, but it doesn't get what's trapped inside of you out. If you want a good fiber choice for later, select a barley fiber, as this is a great source. Psyllium will do too however, just don't think by using a fiber supplement, all your problems are solved. They aren't. What about taking medication? No, drugs are not the answer. Drugs only make you even more toxic. If the body breaths in toxins, if you are eating toxins, if you aren't 'regular' and you aren't getting any healthier, don't you get it?

It is your bowel movements that are limiting the removal of excess waste, cholesterol and toxins. So, let's clean you out. In order to perform an enema properly, the hot water bottle part of your bag must be hung high enough from a rack or wall that the water can flow downward through the hose at a relatively good speed. Pressure is important. It is second in importance to making sure the bag is secure from wherever it hangs so it doesn't fall! And always hang the bag near the toilet. You don't want to fill up with fluids then need to walk very far to let it loose. Once that is in place, you will lay on the floor, on a towel, on your back with your knees bent up and your feet close by your buttocks.

Practice doing a few hip raises from this position. You want to make sure you're situated properly. You want in a stable position where you can raise your hips and shake them up and down a bit with your feet still flat on the floor once the water is inside of you. The combination of warm water, coffee and shaking it all about is what dislodges old decayed feces from inside your intestines and prepares it for excrement. Think of it as shaking a jug full of water to clean it out. It's the same thing.

Once you're full, you will also want to massage your stomach around the abdominal wall muscles, probing deep inside the tissues to 'coax' the fluid through the intestines. This also helps the coffee go higher up inside of you to stimulate the bile release we just discussed. Now, how to fill yourself up... Of course, you will want to lubricate the hose nozzle with oil or a water based lubricant to allow for an easy rectal introduction. Do the same with your anus. Lubricate it. And don't feel funny about it. You are simply taking care of your much neglected health.

In case you fear an entire half gallon bag of water will cause you to explode, there is not only a clip near the end of the nozzle that controls the release of the water to begin with, but most people can hold a full gallon of water without trouble. Just make sure you let a little water run through the hose into the toilet so the air is out of the way before you put the tube inside of you. Once it is in, let the water flow inside of you gently, always controlling the flow using the clip on the hose. Of course there will be some discomfort, bloating, cramps and contractions. It happens until you're cleaned out efficiently.

If the cramps become fierce, simply pause the release of water and relax a moment. Take a deep breath but do not move too quickly during the contraction or you will shoot water all over the place. Poop will certainly follow it! So once the cramps disappear, don't stop the enema, but begin adding more fluid slowly. Eventually, you will be using the whole bag each session. At first, maybe you'll only use a little before you give up, but you still need to come back and do this again anyhow. Not taking a whole bag is just a sign you're full to the rim in there. If someone tells you this process only cleans out the lower intestine, let him or her know two things.

One, a half gallon is too much water to only fill the lower end of your colon. And two, at least your lower end is clean while theirs is still… Well, full of it… You get the picture. You can put it off, but once you begin to realize you're not getting out of this what you put into it, so to speak, I want you to begin doing these enemas daily for 30 straight days. Then, do one every other day for 30 more. After that, do an enema every 3rd day for a month and in the fourth month, just twice a week is good. I would make sure I perform a cleansing once a week after that, usually before bed.

Detoxification IS something of the utmost importance if you want control of your health, let alone your appearance. All of us are toxic and each of us in different amounts. However, the differences between us are: 1) Our individual ability to naturally detoxify ourselves based upon our eating habits. 2) Our total exposure to contaminants and our intake or lack thereof in essential dietary nutrients and 3) Regular hygiene practices that assist in the otherwise sluggish natural cleansing process. Other common symptoms of being toxic include feeling constantly tired, aggravated, or just plain miserable (possibly because you are FAT and BLOATED too, but being overweight is a sure sign of being backed up o matter what you're willing to admit).

Eating right. Is it all about fitness, vanity or health? I spent most of my younger years wanting to attain some very cosmetic goals for myself too. But along the way I saw everyone I knew tearing themselves apart on their quests for a better body. Fitness is the ability to meet the regular demands of your lifestyle more easily and doing so with enough energy left over for the unexpected moments when we really need it. I like being fit. I like eating right and health is something that goes without saying. But maybe we are really just in this for vanity?

Usually that's it and well, I like seeing my knees while looking down towards the floor too. You can only do that if your belly isn't blocking the view. I have said it a million times and I will say it another million times before I die, make health your #1 concern and vanity, your reason for probably being here, will come full circle.

Of the many health challenges that we face daily, problems with the digestive system are the most dangerous and that is why this book focuses on it. Imagine what would be the result if a city's sewer system became so backed up that it actually failed to work at all.

What would happen if sewage pipes got so plugged up that they EXPLODED internally? We wouldn't see what's happening from the outside looking in under most circumstances but it would at least begin to leak gasses and stink. It's not just a bucket of acid in your gut. Some people think if you stick your hand down there, it will be melted within seconds.
Watch the Discovery Channel once in a while. Scientists have been sending little cameras into the human gut and rectum to view the different foods we eat as they get digested. Lord, it's not a good thing to see what is left behind. Take a sandwich for instance. Meats were sometimes visibly left behind when eaten with bread and potatoes. Meat eaten alone however was more often than not, disintegrated to a point it wasn't even there. Hey, the lady who performs our high colonics claims she has never seen foods go through a person as well digested as mine is.

My clients report their technicians state they've never seen people hold as much fluid either. That means we are not only processing our foods but we aren't holding any in our intestines. It's a testimony you may find bizarre but hey, I am not the one with digestive disorders... When you eat your meat with your rice, tell me what you get. GAS. Sometimes AWFUL and foul smelling gas. Gas is indigestion. Undigested foods are what cause gas. In-digestion does not mean you only have a stomach ache per se. IN-digestion means something did NOT completely digest and it is complicating your digestive tract. Ok, so some of you think eating like you do doesn't cause health complications because you do not get headaches, intestinal cramps, bloated, gassed, or whatever, you're OK.

Sorry, you're still deteriorating inside, like it or not, and it's not normal to look the way you do. Sometimes the body shuts off your natural distress warnings like pain signals in your gut because you continue to ignore them. But the cause of those symptoms silently remains. I do my best not to laugh when fat, disgusting, chain smoking, alcoholics or otherwise disturbing people who ignore health criticize me for getting sick if I do. I just nod and ignore them. I can't get mad, and I do feel bad, but sometimes you just got to shake it off. You can't reason with some people. They do not realize if you get sick, that means the body is discarding an illness. It's fighting it off and winning. If you don't get sick, guess what, you are HARBORING the illness. The body is incapable of getting rid of it so it's just sitting in there eating away at your organs. Nice. P.S. When you do get sick, try some PURE honey. It eats away at so many strains of bad bacteria, including the ones not side tracked by antibiotics. Plus it doesn't hurt your good bacteria one bit.

My first enema came as a child when I went to the hospital for constipation. My second came when I returned the next year complaining of belly aches, which the doctor said was just constipation. The next year, I was back in the hospital again for another week's worth of probing. You think that's gross? What do you think the nurses have on their minds when they need to do this for people who won't take care of themselves. A year later my appendix almost burst. The doctor said if I would use fiber and lay off the cup cakes I might not have had that problem. I was only 9 and suffered for 4 years waiting for that advice...

I know you want to be a healthy, vibrant, efficient and productive person. If you are not that type of person currently, odds are you are supporting that lifestyle. Admit it. If I seem intolerant, I am. And I do not feel sorry for you. There is no more time for that and there is no more time for worry, television, or any other waste of energy either. I do not tolerate whiners, excuses, or quitting. Success is from within.

ENSURING YOUR SUCCESS

Take one day each week to figure up what your actual diet was for that past week. Use your average total daily calories from the past seven days to determine what you must schedule for the next seven days. For instance, you may have scheduled 1800 calories a day last week but when you review the entire week when it's all said and done, you might have ended up with more or less here and there day to day. Your average daily intake might actually have been 1700.

Maybe you got fatter this week. I told you not to eat too little or that's what would happen. Maybe you ate 2000 instead of 1800 on the average because you cheated 3 times and that is what made you fat. If you under ate or over ate and got fat, go back and start again at 1800 calories a day for next week. Maybe you ate 2000 calories and made great progress. Stay at 2000 for this week then too. After this, add your calories as suggested each forthcoming week. As we progress, you will notice that you've become more and more tone by building some much needed muscle as you burn off all the unwanted fat (that's how the body is supposed to work).

Once the muscle is built and fat is dropped however, neglecting to feed your new lean body weight is what allows it to disappear and revert back to being fat again. Building muscle speeds the metabolism, losing it slows it down. This is why if you do not eat on time, or eat ENOUGH at ALL times, you become FAT! The body goes into 'ketosis', which is the breakdown of amino acids (muscle protein) for continuous energy. This is what you do to prevent any future headaches... Each week for the first 13 weeks on this program, I want you to ensure progress by adding a few more calories to your diet every seven days. You read that correctly.

Women 5 foot tall generally are able to get down to 100 pounds and remain extremely healthy. However, a good weight for a woman 6 foot tall is 150 pounds. So technically, to determine a good weight for yourself, a woman would add about 4 pounds for every inch over 5 foot tall they are.

So, 5'0" = 100 pounds. But 5'1" = 104, 5'2" = 108, 5'3" = 112, 5'4" = 116, 5'5" = 120, 5'6" = 124, 5'7" = 128, 5'8" = 132, 5'9" = 136, 5'10" = 140, 5'11" = 144, and 6'0" = 148 or so and etc.

Using this scale it will also be obvious what your hips or dress sizes should or should not be at these particular body weights. Ladies, ONLY YOU know your optimal size... And understand, hips aren't what they were at age 17 if you are now 25, 35, 45 or 55. This isn't because of fat, but increased bone density. That's right, brittle bones come from bad habits, not just because you age. Bones are actually supposed to get thicker and stronger as you age but you aren't allowing them to because you've been eating all wrong. Keep this in mind.

Men do well assuming 135 pounds at 5 foot tall and 225 at 6 foot 6 inches is normal. Actually, this may be a little thin for some of you but remember, Bruce Lee was only 135 pounds at 5'7" and Michael Jordan is 216 at 6'6" so you're not far off using this scale. This means to assume a good weight for yourself, add 5 pounds for every inch over 5 foot tall you are to 135 pounds.

So, if you are 5'1" your optimal weight = 140...

5'2" = 145, 5'3" = 150, 5'4" = 155, 5'5" = 160, 5'6" = 165, 5'7" = 170, 5'8" = 175, 5'9" = 180, 5'10" = 185, 5'11" = 190, 6'0" = 195, 6'1" = 200, 6'2" = 205, 6'3" = 210, 6'4" = 215, 6'5" = 220, 6'6" = 225 and so and etc.

A safe waist measure would vary from 29 at 5'0" to 38 inches at 6'6" as well. That's 1 inch larger in waist measurement you are allowed for every 2" taller than 5 foot you are. I am 5'10" which is 10" taller divided by 2 = 5 and so my waist should be 29 inches plus 5 inches = 34" (and it is).

So, if you are 5'1" your waist measure shouldn't be bigger than 29 and a half inches….

5'2" = 30", 5'3" = 30 and a half, 5'4" = 31", 5'5" = 31 and a half, 5'6" = 32", 5'7" = 32 and a half, 5'8" = 33", 5'9" = 33 and a half, 5'10" = 34", 5'11" = 34 and a half, 6'0" = 35", 6'1" = 35 and a half, 6'2" = 36", 6'3" = 36 and a half, 6'4" = 37", 6'5" = 37 and a half, and 6'6" = 38 inches.

Yes, I am certain these figures are accurate. If you weigh the suggested weight and have these waist measures, odds are you are anywhere from 8 to 12% body fat. Some of you are built a little different but guys, like I said to the women, you know if you have an inch to lose or not and you also know if you are over or underweight too. I haven't met you, so you make the call. Point remains, as we progress, you must begin adding calories to maintain your results.

If you are pregnant, wow, you're in luck! You get to add even more food than this! However, keep in mind, while it takes more calories than you're eating when not pregnant in order to create a healthy baby, you do not require all the extra food in one sitting! Pigging out leads to fat babies and no they aren't supposed to be fat! Your child will grow up craving what it was fed in the womb so BE CAREFUL. Do what we just discussed and add only a few extra calories a week gently, as not to overload you or the child. On a weekly basis, over time, simply by adding calories a little as we go, you will feel like a Queen all the way up to welcoming that new addition to your family.

You may start off at 1600 calories a day but by the time Junior comes around, you'll have easily doubled that and kept your body fat levels under control all the while. I understand that as your hormones fluctuate, you may have cravings for the oddest of things. This is only due to a malnourishment of minerals, essential fats or proteins. Other diets, like those that allow for junk foods, deplete you instead of nourish you. Follow these simple instructions and your pregnancy will go much easier and your child will be much healthier.

If you add 50 or 60 calories a week, as long as you supplement with Lemmon's Oil and Multi-Nutrient Formula, you will remain devoid of those cravings, remain fit, not fat, give birth like you rehearsed it a million times already and you will lose the additional weight you gain much easier than anyone else you know. Many women report the delivery process being such a breeze that they almost forgot they even had a baby that day.

If you are starting the diet the day you know you're pregnant and you're currently eating 1500 calories a day, try the following:

Week 1, continue having 1600 calories a day…

Week 2 have 1650 calories a day.

Week 3: 1700.   *Week 4:* 1750.   *Week 5:* 1800.   *Week 6:* 1850.
Week 7: 1900.   *Week 8:* 1950.   *Week 9:* 2000.   *Week 10:* 2050.
Week 11: 2100. *Week 12:* 2150. *Week 13:* 2200. *Week 14:* 2250.
Week 15: 2300. *Week 16:* 2350. *Week 17:* 2400. *Week 18:* 2450.
Week 19: 2500. *Week 20:* 2550. *Week 21:* 2600. *Week 22:* 2650.
Week 23: 2700. *Week 24:* 2750. *Week 25:* 2800. *Week 26:* 2850.
Week 27: 2900. *Week 28:* 2950. *Week 29:* 3000. AND
Week 30, have 3050 calories a day.

Although there are 6 to 9 more weeks left until your child arrives, I cannot recommend that you eat more than this each day. I personally haven't met a woman needing more than 3000 calories a day yet. Who knows, you may be the first, but eat clean. Eat very, very clean. Your baby can get clogged arteries just like you can… After child birth, trim your hips, thighs, belly and butt by cutting back 200 calories a week until you are back down to a couple hundred more calories than you started the diet on. Say if you began at 1600, drop 200 calories a week until you're back down to 1800. Do not drop your calories faster than that, it'll startle your metabolism. Besides, you're healing and nursing.

However, once you're down to that "1800" level, stay there until you visibly tighten up. You will, but be patient and do not make a move without your physician's guidance. For those of you not pregnant, I want you to continue to monitor your waist measurement each week. DON'T SUCK IT IN and pretend you've made progress. Deal with reality. It's so much more exciting. And keep track of everything that you are experiencing on our Know How log sheets. I am not saying everyone 'should' agree with keeping a log book. When things are not working for me, I look at my notes. When things are working well for me, I again look at my notes to see what I am doing correctly. I personally like to know what barriers I have hurdled or what ones I need to approach differently.

You may or may not notice change for the better at first or you may feel like you are definitely heading toward a turn for the worse. If this is the case, re-evaluate your starting point. You probably over estimated your original caloric intake or lied to yourself about how many inches you had to lose to begin with.

Or, if you're right on the money, you may only need to be a little more patient. Wait another week to add more calories. That's not too much to ask is it? Your metabolism is still sluggish, but you will be fine. All that abuse you put your body through over the years takes a little time to reverse folks. Sure you may feel behind schedule and possibly discouraged, but you are learning more and more about your body at the same time. Like all things in life, it's a process. It's also something you should have paid closer attention to long ago. So remain patient and move forward at the you're rate your body allows and learn a little about yourselves along the way.

Men should add 40 to 50 calories a week and women only around 20 to 25. Don't bother trying to divide those calories up to add them a little bit to each meal. 5 or 10 calories here and there are too hard to trace. Do it this way instead:

Week One: Follow your estimated calorie levels.
Week Two: Add calories to your Breakfast.
Week Three: Add calories to your Lunch.
Week Four: Add calories to your Brunch.
Week Five: Add calories to your Mid Day Snack.
Week Six: Add calories to your Dinner.
Week Seven: Add calories to your Breakfast again.
Week Eight: Add calories to your Lunch again.
Week Nine: Add calories to your Brunch again.
Week Ten: Add calories to your Mid Day Snack.
Week Eleven: Add the calories to your Dinner again.
Week Twelve: Add calories to your Breakfast.
Week Thirteen: Add calories to Lunch one more time.

For the majority of you, this is all you'll need and there won't be a worry in the world. The only reason there may be is if you think your muscle mass is more than it really is to begin with.

If you are worried about what results to expect and think progress is based on particular body structures, STOP. Don't worry. You're not that different than anybody else. It's simple. An 'ecto' morph is a thin person. A 'meso' morph is a medium sized person. An 'endo' morph is a bigger person. None of this really matters though in regards to your progress or what routine to follow unless you want to have a boring conversation with someone else trying to sound smart. I am explaining it only because many before you have enquired about it. Using Greek terms to describe things like body composition and musculature is silly in the scope of simply tossing the correct foods down your neck for a change. All you need to know about losing fat and building muscle you've already read today.

To build muscle, you must drop body fat. To drop body fat you must build muscle. To accomplish this, some need to eat less. Some need to eat more. Knowing much of anything else really doesn't matter. Only your eating habits matter. When you get someone who is underweight on this diet, they are automatically going to GAIN muscular weight without getting fat. If you get somebody who is currently overweight on this diet, that person is going to start losing weight in the form of fat. It's the natural process the body follows when properly nourished. But you MUST eat enough…

I was told at age 16 by our family physician when I was wanting to gain weight that I was an 'ecto' morph and would never weigh more than 150 pounds. That's funny because when I was born, I was 10 pounds and the doctor said I was an 'endo' morph who was going to be a beast in size by adulthood. I weighed 108 when I was 16. I weighed 150 a little while later at age 17. Eventually I was 274 and drug free when I took up bodybuilding.

So I hardly think your current bone size makes much of a difference. Only your diet does.

CHEATING AND CHEAT DAYS

What about cheating (as in mixing your foods INCORRECTLY)? People don't realize that when they are about to cheat on something that it has a healthier alternative. The desire to cheat should be read as a specific signal from the body as something other than the obvious. Some people reach for potato chips, others reach for candy. One craving is for sugar, and the other is not for salt but for minerals. Some crave steak. That's a protein craving.

Each and every one of us has different cravings and each of them are different signals. If you crave proteins, have something healthy with protein in it. If you crave salty food, get some green vegetables in you. If you crave sugar, you are really in need of essential fats. Foot the bill and you'll fit into your favorite clothing in no time. Revert back to your old eating habits and I cannot be held accountable. As long as you can determine whether what you want is a fat, a protein or a carbohydrate food, you can literally continue to eat anything and scare that craving away.

With the exception of what you already know is bad for you, practically anything is allowed. If you want to have something you can't avoid mixing incorrectly (even though there are sugar or fat free versions available of anything you could possibly imagine these days) do so at only that one meal (IF you need to do that at all). Actually, I insist you cheat every now and then on whatever it is you may want. It will teach you a lesson you wouldn't learn otherwise. I feel like a sloppy pig when I eat badly. I get gas that scares the neighbors. I get headaches and am a bear to be around. But it's your choice. Live how you want. If you do cheat, even by accident or in the event of an emergency because it was between deciding to starve or… Whether to eat anything you can get your hands on (which is rare), pull your car over, buy a burger at a fast food joint, throw the bun out or run to the grocery store for fruit, nuts or cold cuts. In the future, always have food and water packed to travel with you nearby. And when you have something you probably shouldn't, don't go overboard. Try to stay within your calorie range for the meal anyhow and resume the program on schedule like nothing ever happened (forget that you ever cheated) afterwards. Whatever the case is, do not skip the next meal just because you feel guilty. Take complete responsibility for the consequences of your own actions, learn from them and climb back on the wagon. Blowing one meal is no big deal.

Skipping a meal is! If you cheat, you set yourself back a day. If you skip a meal, you set yourself back another day. When eating out you cannot control the serving sizes you receive, so remember that you are not obligated to clean your plate. Ask for a doggy bag. If you aren't sure what to get when out with friends, I find ordering only meat and steamed veggies with a side salad but no croutons always works. If you ask for a little butter and Caesar's dressing to dip your fork in to take bites from your salad, no one will think you're eating weird.

I avoid anything Alfredo, battered, breaded, creamed, crisped, or deep-fried like they contain a plague because Lord only knows what all is in these dishes. Seize control of your dining decisions. Let nothing and no one stand in your way. I know some diets are much more lenient. The reason those other programs advocate cheating or even eating more foods on weekends is because those diets want you to take longer to reach your goals. Seriously. If you cheat, you get fat. You get fat, you go out and buy more of their products and stay on their systems even longer. It's actually brilliant from a marketing perspective.

However, this only leads to personal failure, low self-esteem, a lot of wasted time, frustration, enclosure, dead ends, harbored emotions, and a fat, sloppy looking body. Do you know why people you admire most never seem to fail? They don't quit. The definition of "failure" is "quitter." Talent is not their secret.

There are, granted, many keys to success and talent may be one of them, BUT this "know how" is an "education" that leads towards "understanding." Your ability to understand is based upon your desire to become educated. Desire IS based upon determination. Determined people are disciplined through education to succeed by the best means possible.

However, successful people CREATE their talent. If you self-discipline yourself, you will not be intimidated by anything between you and the desire of reaching your goals. That takes something beyond talent and education. It takes patience. Sure, you'll make some mistakes and there will be roadblocks but pay attention to them. Roadblocks and mistakes are merely opportunities from which you can gain greater knowledge. Higher learning. Better understanding. Everything you do in life is a chance to become more talented. You will learn things you need to succeed instead of fail if you walk patiently forward in life. Things I can't personally teach you are gained from experience.

This particular experience is RE-CREATION-AL, as in FUN-creating, or creating fun and it is not so much 'work' after all. You'll like this. But some of you will quit anyways. You will not only fail, but learn, therefore understand, succeed or solve ANYTHING for yourself. Nor will you gain talent. Worrying about this only puts off solving the problem, moving forward. There has never been a single thing solved through worry. Worrying, is in fact, so NOT right, it's totally WRONG. I understand that occasionally people aren't trying to be stubborn, or hard headed. They sincerely don't understand all that is laid before them. Well, let me be the first to tell you something else… YOU DO NOT NEED TO UNDERSTAND MOST THINGS IN LIFE TO PUT THE EFFORT INTO MOVING FORWARD.

So welcome back to REALITY. Put your issues and everything else negative behind you. It's time to move forward. "If you think you can, or if you think you can't, you are absolutely right."

Believe in yourself. Don't drive yourself nuts thinking life's little pleasures are gone for good and this isn't going to be any fun. How long is the wait? Well, first, get to your goal. Why would you want to do anything that prevents you from getting to where you want to be safely without any headaches?

Once you succeed, say when you can see your stomach muscles, you can cheat, but only on specific days. How old are you? At the time I wrote this I was 30, so I cheat only once every 30 days. Are you 53? You could realistically cheat every 53 days then. The older you get, the more sensitive your digestive system becomes (like sewage pipes, they go bad in time, only yours can't be replaced, so keep them healthy). A 16 year old could cheat almost every other week. Allowing for more than that is exactly why you haven't gotten where you have liked or struggled to get there if you have. I know some diets are much more lenient.

The reason some diets advocate cheating is because it sets you back and you'll stay on their program longer and longer buying more and more of their products as you go . You really don't have to cheat at all if you do not want to. But go ahead, it's OK. I said you could. If you are going crazy, once a week sounds fine if you are in good shape already, but I just want you to take care of YOURSELF. If you crave carbs, have protein. If you crave salts, have carbs, but only have good clean sources of these foods if you want to remain on track. Once a month I used to get a slice of peanut butter pie from the Hard Rock Café. They no longer serve it. I went 2 years until I had that pie again but it was at the Winking Lizard in Independence, Ohio. That is the only thing I can remember wanting in years. I still want a piece, but I do not CRAVE ONE and THAT is the difference…

Media hype may tell us Jennifer Lopez's big butt is supposed to be attractive. She's pretty, but that butt isn't. Society also tells us music groups that do not write their own songs are talented. Kids believe they do. Next week they will tell us something different. Step away from it all. Do not use what 'everyone says' or 'knows' as a gauge for what YOU should believe in or do.

Tip: For those of you investing in CLA and HMB at your local health food store, consider this, CLA and HMB can be obtained for pennies on the dollar by eating 2 tablespoons of raw cream and just 1 tablespoon of real butter a day.

All cream and dairy fat contains CLA (a fat that regulates hormones). It's 0.1 to 0.5% of the total fat. If nothing else, that beats paying the $40 a bottle at a health food store for CLA supplements.

NATURAL ENERGY PRODUCTION

The hesitation people actually have with food separation is iron-ically due to their thinking this is a low carbohydrate plan believe it or not. Yeah, of all things. Because I only suggest 2 carb meals a day, people think this is a low carb plan. They think they will tire out with only two carb meals, especially during a workout. There are two types of exercise. One is aerobic or 'cardiovascular' exercise, and the other is 'anaerobic' weight (resistance) training. As far as nutrition goes, there isn't much of a difference.

Aerobic athletes do tend to require an extra carb meal on marathon days but they could also use an extra protein meal. Competitive weight lifters or bodybuilders also require an extra carb meal after their training sessions, but they too, like anyone else, require only 2 carb meals on off days. Plan your schedule accordingly but I do not care who you are, track athletes, or the general fitness folks, we are all alike in one way and that is you require 4 protein and 2 carb meals a day typically.

First of all, the misconception that you must receive all your energy via glycogen, glucose and carbohydrates is incorrect. And despite it being considered the most logical idea to reduce carbs to lose fat, it is another myth that you need to eliminate carbohydrates altogether from your diet in order to burn body fat. All you have to do is 'reduce' them, not eliminate them. Low carbohydrate or 'ketogenic' diets are hazardous. Did you know being in a constant state of ketosis means your body is not adapting correctly to your diet? It is actually a sign that it has begun breaking itself down.

Despite the fact that they say the hormones released while on a low carb plan (glucocorticoids and glucagon) mobilize the liver's reserve of glycogen (carbs), so you burn fat, that's not exactly how it works. Keeping the liver low in carbohydrates for efficiency reasons is one thing, but the muscles are the next thing to be burnt and you don't want that to happen. You will fall flat (which always happens once your muscle glycogen is lost). Anyways, this isn't a low carb diet.

I want you to eat carbs twice a day without fail. This is a decrease for some of you and an increase for others. Adjusting your carbohydrate intake slightly either way will not adversely affect you if you also increasing your essential fatty acids. This is because good fats work well with protein. Carbs do not. And while carbs might interfere with other metabolic processes or deplete you of minerals whereas fats do not, you won't be eating that many carbs if you only have them twice a day.

In regards to the idea following other diets that in order to use proteins properly you need to eat them with carbs, having carbs at every meal only makes you carb dependent, and a sugar addict. Sure, you can always do 60 minutes of aerobics twice a day, mix your foods, and stay fairly lean if you eat low fat, but that's like racing your truck uphill with a trailer hitched on the back. Instead you should be driving a much efficient vehicle that runs on better fuel to get the job done easier. Almost any vehicle will get you to the top, but one doesn't force you to work so hard nor wonder if you're ever actually going to make it to the top at all.

I choose the high performance vehicle. Either way, a carbohydrate dependent body is NOT a good thing. The body's attempt to produce most of its energy from carbohydrates is why you cramp and burn during exercise. It is from the buildup of lactic acid that high carb intakes produce. Do you lie awake sleepless at night or get cramps that are almost unbearable? That's from either having too many sugars in your diet or even worse, a lack of the nutrients which prevent the cramping.

If you are getting what you feel is enough nutrition but you still cramp, you may want to look into the type of carbohydrate you ingest or the quality of the products you use. Alcoholics get cramps all the time by the way. Alcohol depletes minerals....

Marketing hype may have you believing you need carbs for their sugars in order to transport your proteins but no matter what this simply isn't true. The body eventually turns everything you eat into one form of sugar or another (and ultimately all sugar gets turned into various forms of alcohol before it is entirely processed) and that includes proteins and fats. Sure, you can argue that you need all three nutrients in lesser or equal values as per the Zone diet but I beg to differ the rationale.

When glucose enters the bloodstream after the digestion of carbohydrates, proteins or fats, insulin eventually gets secreted by the pancreas to utilize them. From there, the next step is going to be either good or bad based upon the nutrients currently available inside of you or what you just ate. If you ate too much carbohydrate food for instance, it cannot and will not be stored as glycogen even if there are sufficient nutrients and enzymes available in the bloodstream to do so. There is only 'so much' room to store all the carbs you eat in your liver or muscles, folks.

The excess causes a depletion of other vital nutrients to get rid of it and either ends up wasted or stored as fat. Either way, YOU lose, but it depends on what condition you have yourself in right now and what you ate with those carbs that make the difference. The excess or unusable carbohydrates are usually transferred into a form of triglycerides before they are stored as body fat. If you ate fat at this meal with those carbs, guess where that goes once the excess carbs are stored as fat? You guessed it. Around your butt and gut. Birds of a feather flock together my friend. Eventually, when there is a need for more energy that the diet doesn't supply, stored glycogen is, yes, converted back into glucose and used by cells or transported through the bloodstream for further conversion and use.

But this only happens during exercise or starvation (which is what low carb diets do… They STARVE you). And even if it is during exercise and not because you are starving, once glycogen is depleted, you will not enter into what you think is a fat burning zone. What? Why not? Well, you see, glycogen is in limited availability when it comes to energy. It can deplete in as little as 10 to 15 minutes under extreme conditions. Ever worked real hard for 10 straight minutes and began shaking? You depleted yourself of glycogen.

Yes, that quickly. And once it's gone, the body demands that it is immediately replaced or what you think is your fat burning zone actually results in muscle degeneration. This doesn't mean you need more carbohydrates during the exercise session. The body doesn't digest and react that quickly even with simple sugars. Carbohydrates, while they are quick energy sources, were not meant to be your primary source of energy. You need dietary fat for that. No? Then why do the experts say glycogen only lasts you about 20 to 30 minutes MAXIMUM during exercise?

Why do physicians say you burn more muscle than fat once it is gone? Because carbs are meant for short bursts of energy and fat is meant for longer-term use. Before we go any further, it is this depletion of glycogen that is PRECISELY why your exercise sessions must be shortened as well. More on that later. Let's continue. We can solve all of your problems by simply eating fat with protein PRIOR to your workouts. In doing this you are signaling to the body that you want it to protect its glycogen because you are giving it something else to burn. Once it runs out of dietary fat, the body will then begin to BURN BODY FAT during the session leaving the protein alone.

What if the preferred energy source to begin with always was fat? Carbs fill the muscle and organs and then protein builds and heals tissues. You see, the body only uses carbs when it runs low on fat to burn. Then once it runs out of carbs, you'll always burn muscle before anything else. The body then goes scavenging for more and more carbs as replacement. Remember this because without proper fat in the diet, once you run low on glycogen, the body breaks protein down for glucose and you'll continually struggle to make progress. IMAGINE THE RESULTS if you take advantage of what I have just said.

I used to have plain tasting pure whey mixed with filtered water, whole cream and ginger before my workouts but I can no longer find a good source of whey from anyone who hasn't 'sold out' and corrupted their product. Since I have gotten fine results on the coffee and cream alone. Then afterwards I have something like a bagel with raisins or another carb. This is a virtually fool proof method that reverses a number of negative mechanisms happening internally that can cause you to feel drained, exhausted, aggravated, fatigued, and etc if you do not do pay attention. Even if you do not understand, you WILL AT LEAST recover faster from your training this way.

And recovery from working out, despite the other stresses of everyday living, is what allows for progress. How is that possible? Well, it is still recommended that you eat carbs separate from your proteins. But once food digests, it enters your bloodstream. This is what elevates your blood sugar levels or the amount of protein available inside of your body. What occurs next is actually a constant lingering of available glucose or amino acids that's still available when you eat one or two of your following meals. This is the reason why we have protein meals before our workouts and save the carbohydrates for afterwards. I know it is the opposite that most experts suggest but protein digests slowly, carbs digest faster.

So if you eat your protein now, in about 2 hours once it has digested, the amino acids from that protein meal will then be just about ready and waiting in your bloodstream to start healing your sore muscles. If you eat carbs at the correct times, like just as soon as the workout is over, then the glucose will enter the system in time to assist the protein to your tissues for recovery. Those same carbs will also still be around for the benefit of your next couple of meals if you eat enough (but not too much mind you). If you eat carbs at the wrong times, like before a workout, you'll end up fat...

Does that make it simple enough to understand? It is what you eat now, that makes food work better for you when you eat again later... That covers your workouts, muscle building, fat burning, etc. But in everyday life, there are still three basic steps in the production of energy whether it comes through fat, protein or carbohydrate metabolism. We know that once any food is eaten it is turned to glucose or sugar and those three steps by which it's done are glycolysis, the citric acid cycle (CAC or Kreb's cycle) and the electron transport chain (ETC).

The net result of the entire production is something called ATP (adenosine tri-phosphate). ATP is the energy source of just about everything we do. It is an organic chemical compound that acts like a converter, controlling the power switches that keeps us alive. ATP is constantly being manufactured, stored, and burned 24 hours a day. Chronic fatigue is one of the most common problems plaguing society today, second only to obesity and a lack of ATP explains why. You see, of the food we eat, almost half of it is supposed to keep our metabolism going. The other half is supposed to provide energy in the form of ATP.

The process of manufacturing ATP is known as oxidative phosphorylation, which is merely the coupling of phosphorus and adenosine. But before we can even begin to worry about this, we need to understand that carbohydrates may not be the best fuel in initiating the phosphorylation process. Glycosis and CAC provide the groundwork for the ETC process. Luckily, Glycolysis can generate the CAC from whatever you eat. However, when it is produced from carbohydrates, because they burn so fast, there is very little raw material left over to perform the third and most crucial step, the building of that electron transport chain (ETC).

The first step for fat metabolism however is beta-oxidation, which yields 2 carbon groups for the citric acid cycle to function. An amino acid's (protein molecule's) first step is de-amination, a process where the amino acids are removed from the protein by the liver and the kidneys. That means fat and protein burn a little slower than carbs do and as we know with all other things, the more careful nature is adhered to, the more efficient you become. Efficiency in this case results in a faster metabolism and more natural energy. No more coffee, no more fatigue.

There's never a lack of energy on this program unless you subject yourself to a lack of sleep, water or food. If you have been following the program but aren't seeing results, then you aren't really 'on' the program. This is precisely why I insist you send your diet to me whenever it changes for re-cvaluation. We cannot guarantee you understand everything and are 'on' the 'diet' unless I see with my own two eyes. It's easy to misunderstand something considering my ideas are so radical and new to you. If you send me your daily routine to look at, I will fix everything for you. I promise.

I need to know your name, age, height, weight, and what you eat and drink at all your meals. From there, we will get you on track. As good as this is beginning to sound, simply eating protein and fat together isn't enough if you continue to insist on a low calorie, low carb, and low fat diet. That puts you in a state of serious ketosis (remember, that's muscle burning for energy, and not a good thing). But if sufficient calories are available and enough fat is present, you are safe from muscle wasting. Just how much protein and fat? More of both, especially if you haven't been eating much of either.

Calorie restrictive diets don't work because they remove as much muscle as they do fat and that only makes you look fatter although you look smaller. Muscle is the only engine that burns fat. The more muscle you lose, the less fat you burn. What happens if you haven't had fat in a while? When fat is reintroduced to your diet (even just a little), and carbs are reduced or increased to just two meals a day, most of your energy will almost immediately come from the breakdown of fatty acids.

Initially it will be from the dietary fat but eventually, that unsightly stored body fat will diminish as the cycle continues (which takes from 3 to 7 weeks to fully experience results, you'll know why in a minute) too. The body will not store the fat we suggest you eat. The body only stores fat because either you eat too many carbs, mix your foods incorrectly or you limit fat intake. And we aren't suggesting you eat a lot of fat. We are simply recommending that you add the right fats back into your diet. If you do this and maintain it, the enzymes that break fat down will prevent you from ever becoming overweight again.

Basically, a diet a little higher in fat, activates the lipolytic (fat burning) enzymes in your body and decreases the activity of the lipogenic (fat producing) enzymes. A body which receives too much fat reacts much the same way a body with too many carbohydrates would. You get fat from it. So stick with that 3 to 1 protein to fat gram ratio I recommended in the 12 Food Groups for 4 meals and have carbs at two other meals and you'll be fine.

Now you know, certain other metabolic pathways are blocked if you eat a lot of carbohydrates. The body won't efficiently make energy from glucose, nor use proteins or fats correctly if this happens. This is the theory that conned so many of you to try the Zone. What kept it from working was the same thing that kept anything else from working, the food separation. The result of all those other plans was a continued craving of glucose (sugar) for glycolysis, right? What do you think is going on when we get noticeably drowsy after eating a lot of carbs after you binge? A moderate, or reduced, carb intake prevents drowsiness and binging. Simply reduce or increase your intake to only 2 carb meals a day as soon as possible.

If you go with less or try more right now, depending on what you are used to doing, you will burn out, fatigue, and confuse the other tissues that will then start trying to replace lost carbs... That again means losing muscle. Subsequently, if you won't heed this advice, hypoglycemia will develop and this stresses not only the adrenal glands but your pancreas. What did we learn today? Carbohydrates are essential to maintaining internal sugar stores, but using them as your primary energy source is like using one lamp to light up an entire house. It doesn't work and your entire system is thrown for a loop. When we run low and we ingest more carbohydrates to replace what is lost, this only 'fuels' us with just 'enough' energy. Forget hypoglycemia or diabetes, hypo-adrenia eventually develops (a state in which your adrenal system becomes stressed trying to pick up the resulting slack you have caused).

This is what I meant when I said you not only get tired, but it's also why you get irritable sometimes after you eat. Two carb meals a day are all you need to stay within the 'too much' or 'too little' ZONE. Just try it. You may not be sure either way what is right. That's why I am here.

To tell you what actually works. It does a lot of good by thinking of carbs as a secondary energy source and EATING more fat than you have in the past. I emphasize this AGAIN, because the body will, under most conditions, take muscle protein and turn it into a form of glucose (via gluconeogenesis) for energy once carbohydrates are exhausted if and essential fatty acids aren't there. Trust me on this. A good analogy to describe ATP use is like comparing the process to an average every day battery. Batteries get overused to a point that all it's capable of producing is unusable fizzles.

Rechargeable batteries that can have energy put back in them can also only perform again if it is replenished first. ATP then is like the higher energy source, the rechargeable battery. ADP is the lesser energy source or a drained battery. ATP becomes ADP if it isn't recharged in time and that's when the body depletes itself looking for something that isn't there to turn itself back into ATP. This is likened to tossing your belongings out of a closet blindly behind you looking for a needle. Everything goes into disarray and takes quite a while to clean before anything is operating normally again. Let's try to avoid this the best we can.

First thing you should do right now is show this book to your friends if any of them know anything about biochemistry. Get their feedback. Call a professional. See what they say. One thing is for certain, if you soak this all in, your life is about to change. Those around you need to know why and how. Do not keep it a secret you used this program and make sure you can tell them WHY your changes occurred. Of course read the rest of the book first so you can talk the talk after walking the walk.

And by finishing the book first, you'll know why you are experiencing all the negative things that you are these days. If you think the answer lies in an exercise plan, then why hasn't exercise achieved all your goals for you yet? Just keep them in order and once you've gotten through the entire book, send me those questions. Many times my views challenge the supposedly educated and well researched people who figure if they didn't know something already, no one else could either. I am here to help you and I will, despite the fact you are in denial. I am willing to help the most stubborn of you to get on the right path. But remain patient and finish the book first.

ESSENTIAL VS COMMERCIAL FATS

This next section is for those of you who require more informa-tion as to why fats are so important before you will try them. If you do not add at least one tablespoon of the right (essential) fats a day, NO other supplements you use will fully benefit you NOR will your food digest properly NOR will anything else you do regarding health, work in your favor. If you use lotion for dry skin or your kid uses pimple cream for acne, all they need is some essential fatty acids. Not eating real oil because you are taking only capsules? That is another reason why you're having these problems.

Capsules are made by heating oil. Heated oil is dead. Without fresh, unheated, raw essential fatty acids, little by little, every-thing in your entire body eventually fails. No? I haven't met a woman yet who eats a low fat diet that doesn't experience degenerative reproductive system disorders (like not having a period). I haven't met a man yet who eats a low fat diet that doesn't end up with a low sperm or testosterone count. In fact, I had a couple of friends who were smokers and couldn't have a child no matter how hard they tried for the better part of over 10 years. They blamed the smoking. I did too in part because smoking depletes the nutrients essential fats normally try to pro-tect inside of you.

His wife didn't smoke as much, but she did smoke sometimes. And since the husband's family were all chain smokers, she suf-fered from more second hand smoke than anyone else I had ever known. And to top it off, she was following a low fat diet to 'maintain' her figure. Her hubby was a baker and ate so many pastries that I couldn't even begin to assume how much hydrogenated oil was clogging his veins...

However, even with all this, after just 30 days of taking the essential oil I recommended, she became pregnant. For 10 years, they had nothing. After 4 weeks and 2 days of essential oils, there was a baby on the way. Coincidence? No. She quit taking the supplements after 60 days and lost the baby. Her physician told her that whatever she did to clean up her system over those first 30 days should have been continued. After just 30 days off the supplements, her blood work improved and went back to what it was months before. A baby couldn't form under those conditions.

No, these two people weren't fitness competitors, athletes or models. But now that I have your attention, I want to go a bit more in depth so you can understand how essential fatty acids affect all of us. Fats really are the single most important nutrients we require although they only account for 10% of the 100 essential nutrients. Fat regulates your hormones. Fat also kills your hormones. Fat carries vitamins and minerals to your cells in order to nourish you and if you miss out on taking in enough essential fats on a daily basis, you not only lose out on 10% of what your overall success may be, but you lose out on 33% of what goes on inside of you because the other nutrients and even your organs can't function without them. Over time, this adds up to nothing but trouble.

For example, we mentioned earlier how the liver normally puts excess cholesterol in bile. Well, it is supposed to send it to the gall bladder, which then empties it into the small intestine just below the stomach for excretion. It cannot do this if you're only eating olive oil and cup cakes. It clogs and becomes backed up on a 'normal' diet. You must realize that the removal of excess cholesterol and waste is a natural process that we must accommodate with proper nutrition. If not, we experience elevated cholesterol levels in the blood and disease.

That's right, what I am trying to tell you is that the right kind of fats regulate cholesterol and reverse high blood pressure. Bad fats do not. It's a fact. And essential fats do not make you fat like bad fat does. The body instantly recognizes them as 'good' for you and puts them to use for healing and growth as soon as you ingest them. The difference is that you have to ingest these fats. The body doesn't make essential fats on it's own and they are not contained in things found at the grocery store. Therefore we supplement….

Here is why. There are several kinds of fats, and two are essential (EFA): Omega 3 (n-3 or w3) and Omega 6 (n-6 or w6). All other fats, such as omega 9 (mono-unsaturated), omega 7, and the saturated fats, are non-essential because the body CAN produce these ones quite easily from sugars and starches if need be. Good fats regulate immune and inflammatory responses, lower risk factors for cardiovascular disease, reduce high triglycerides, and even improve your vision. The opposite is true of 'bad' fats. Omega 3's and Omega 6's are good fats. Omega 9 fats are neutral, so to speak. The important thing to remember is that essential fats must be taken in the right amounts, in proper ratios, just like the suggested RDA percent of vitamins and minerals if we want the best results. Where do we get them?

Usable Omega 6 fats are found in sesame, flax or sunflower seeds and most nuts. Animal meats and many fish sources contain the Omega 6 derivative arachidonic acid (AA) which, while a little different, are just as important as the Omega 6's found in nuts and seeds. Sources of Omega 3's are found in flaxseeds and green leafy vegetables but that's not the same Omega 3 that comes from cold-water fish such as albacore tuna, Atlantic halibut, salmon and shellfish. The problem with fish sources though is that it is almost impossible to ingest enough to supply the fats sufficiently.

This is because of the abundance of essentials needed to meet the body's requirements daily. But we can't give up now! We really do need to get these fats from somewhere. Our brain alone is over 60% fat, and EFA's are vital components to not only the brain but the rest of the nervous system. In fact, if mothers become depleted of EFA's during pregnancy, their children's optimal spine development is limited. As we already discussed, it is common for malnourished women, even those who think they are nourished, to lose their babies. It is well known that EFA's are necessary for every cell's growth from the moment of conception to the day we die.

The common malnourishment we all share began with something that happened in 1900. This is when a different type of fat appeared in our diets. That fat has increased in availability by about 20 times since then. This fat is derived from a particular form of vegetable oil. How can we avoid it? That's hard to say. We are unwittingly eating these bad fats even when we think we are eating 'right.' So, it's no wonder your health has degenerated and you can't get into shape as easy as you would like.

Couple getting bad fats in your health foods with the 'low' fat, 'no' fat, and 'fake' fat diets that have been further depriving people of the good stuff and we've got a lot of work ahead of us if we want to get our health back. So, as of this moment, you need to make the conscious decision to cut out junk food if you want your cholesterol under control. Even 'partially' hydrogenated oils like margarine, although cholesterol free, are bad. Sure, butter (and egg yolks too) contain cholesterol, but they also contain natural fat mobilizing nutrients. When foods are eaten in their own whole food form, they are more than able to metabolize themselves. Margarines do not have this going for them.

Margarines are fake fats made by taking an otherwise 'good' cis-linoleic acid and adding a hydrogen to the double bonds which turns them into un-natural forms of saturated fats in a Frankenstein-ish 'trans' formation. This is done so they last longer on a store shelf and for no other reason. This is unfortunate because you try to eat fat free foods or health food bars and protein powders but only have your blood cholesterol escalate beyond your control. Drop these un-natural fats and foods containing them from your diet and you will have your 'bad' LDL cholesterol levels return to normal quite rapidly (whether or not the genetic tendency runs high in your family).

It isn't genetics which raise your cholesterol. It's your everyday HABITS. The Harvard School of Public Health has warned us for years on the dangers of eating margarines, commercially baked snack goods, and deep fried foods as opposed to using good fats like real butter, extra virgin olive oil (means the olive hasn't fallen from the tree before processing) and Omega 3 fats because it's the processed oils that are making us die slow, painful deaths. Many of those who listened have turned to unre-fined flax oil, which is high in omega 3, thinking this will help solve their problem. It doesn't always help.

Using flax oil alone can disrupt the natural balance of things and lead to a shortage of omega 6 fats if you aren't careful. Fats (triglycerides, cholesterols, phospholipids, etc) all pro-duce the precursors to your hormones, tissues and cells. Including the ones for creating either fat loss, muscle growth, normal development or having a baby (from a man or a woman's perspective). But in order to understand why you need such a balance, we need a more in-depth discussion on the GOOD vs. BAD fats. Good fats act as anti-oxidants, anti-inflammatory agents.

They even produce fat burning enzymes. However, you MUST ingest a fat called gamma linolenic acid to activate your 'good' brown fat cells to burn away your ugly 'white' fat cells. Borage oil and primrose oil are good sources of this one. Do you remember me saying that cholesterol is actually a required nutrient? (You get 90 milligrams or so with every 3 ounces of meat you eat.) Well, it regulates your every cell so that actually makes it a good fat. You need it daily. No two ways about it. In fact, under most conditions, two thirds of the cholesterol that is inside of you is produced by the body itself and only a third of it is actually derived from the food you eat.

There are only two explanations for having high or elevated cholesterol. Either you are producing too much of it for some reason (possibly a backed up liver) or you are eating too much of it to begin with (which is only a problem if your body isn't breaking it down). Another good fat is alpha linolenic acid (ALA) which produces the acids that limit the growth of 'bad' hormones, so that's obviously helpful. You can get ALA from walnuts, flax seed, and other cold weather oils. We're not done yet. On top of this, you still need 6 grams per 100 pounds you weigh of linoleic acids. That's about a half tablespoon.

Note: I know it's confusing because some acids are spelled or sound nearly the same as others but they are NOT the same type of fats. And remember, 1000 milligrams of any type of fat equals 1 full gram in measure and a gram of fat contains 9 calories each. This is important because studies throughout the years have shown that 6% of your diet should consist of these essential fatty acids alone. Yet, even more has proven beneficial when it comes to maintaining lower blood fat levels and inhibiting arterial plaque. If you are on a low fat diet, half your fat should be from essentials.

However, if you are on a low carb diet, you will need an extra 4 grams of Omega 3 fish oils (EPA and DHA) combined with a teaspoon of flax seed oil (works synergistically together) to keep your mental acuity straight. DHA (found in both oils) is SO essential that without it, your mind degenerates and you will actually burn brain cells. The reason we mix the two instead of selecting just one is because the Omega 3 fatty acids found in flax seed and walnuts (50% of the flax seed is Omega 3 while walnut oil has only 20%) are totally different sources than Omega 3's from fish. In fact, fish liver oil Omegas are good for night blindness but seed oil Omega 3's are better for renal damage.

This means if you have kidney stones you will not benefit from fish liver oil. But you will from the seed source of oil while very similar, they are different. You must also be careful not to ingest spoiled, over processed, rancid and toxic fat sources. (if it smells like fish, it's spoiled.) Many sources of oils and fish products are. Only fresh oils work. You may as well seal your own coffin taking the oils most outlets supply you. I will tell you where to get your oils in a bit. You now see we need many different kinds of fats. Some are necessary, some we can burn, some we store and some that poison us. Out of all of this, there are really only three that affect us. The differences between the three lie the reason we need to receive these fats in balanced amounts.

Most aging afflictions like heart attacks, strokes, arthritis, and headaches or symptoms such as graying hair, wrinkles, etc… are all related to what we have just discussed so far. Preventative measures must be taken today to protect you 30 years from now, however, I repeat, simply chugging down some flax seed oil isn't going to do the trick.

Every fat we eat, no matter the source, is eventually converted into more specific hormones called prostagladins (PG for short). There are PG1, PG2 and PG3 groups. Groups 1 and 3 are the good hormones, PG2's are the bad guys, at least in the hormone world. PG1 and 3's control blood clots, pressure, swelling, inflammation, and tumors. PG2's do the opposite. PG2's cause dis-ease. PG1's are from fats found in safflower, sunflower, primrose and currant oils. They are Omega 6's. PG1's require several biochemical changes and are dependent upon di-homo-gamma-linolenic acid (DGLA) to butterfly into good hormones.

PG1's are slow and tedious in making this transition process. It takes time to get things right. As for the elderly, this PG1 process is ever important as these particular hormones are the ones which carry calcium and other minerals into your bones and tissues instead of pulling them out like the bad fats do. Get these good fats under control and calcium deposits will become a thing of the past. The other good hormones, the PG3's, are made from fats found in walnut, flax and cold-water fish oils (Omega 3's).

They require but one biochemical change in becoming a hormone from a fat. Reason being, they are equipped with their own "Omega 3 exclusive" EPA (ei-co-sa-pent-ae-no-ic) acid enzyme. It is well known in medical circles that PG3 hormone stimulating fats are fat burning and illness fighting heroes. These fats are good for men looking to raise their testosterone, women to maintain their femininity and even cancer or AIDS patients trying to build their white blood cells. PG2's however, the bad guys, come not only from the fats in red meats, shell fish (neither of these sources are really so bad) but they are ESPECIALLY BAD if they come from hydrogenated oils and fake fats (OH SO VERY BAD).

These fats only require one step instead of several to change into hormones like the PG3's do. Because PG2 fats process the fastest of all the PG's, leaving PG1 and 3's at a biochemical disadvantage, PG2's poison you long before the good guys are around to help you! The Catch 22 occurred when we discovered some of the naturally occurring fats (like stearic acid, which is necessary for a normal metabolism) such as though found in meat and shell fish that breed PG2's. You see, we can have a little PG2 in our system and be safe, but the PG2's that come from oil sources (oils that never spoil) like hydrogenated coconut, palm and baking oils are the problem.

It is key to point out that the arachidonic acids that all fats eventually become are dependent of their own built in enzymes. Arachidonic acid (AA) is NOT found in these commercially accepted oils and lards. AA is needed to break down the stearic acid (which we mentioned earlier is necessary for a normal metabolism) in our animal fats, but since it isn't there to do this in processed fats, we have a problem. This lack of AA is the link that leads to blocking the conversion of PG1 and 3's into good (life saving) hormones. Again, because animal fats have this component, they are safe. It is foods like creamy peanut butter, commercial snack foods and French fries you need to avoid.

Those foods contain fake fats, hydrogenated oils, and trans-fatty acids that are NOT acceptable by any means. Meat is alright. Get it now? Sure, you should limit your animal fat intake (by trimming your steak marbles, shedding the skin off your chicken, tossing out a few egg yolks, etc), but do not limit your animal protein sources. Protein assists PG1 and 3's in doing their jobs and converting into healthy hormones! I know, I know, I know, you love your peanut butter. So do I! In it's natural form, peanut butter is fine.

But after it is processed, creamed, hydrogenated and then having had sugar added to it, it's now B-A-D. Here is why. Hydrogenated fats (lards) in addition to sugar, alcohol, smoking, stress, toxicity, low protein diets and many other factors all block the enzyme delta 6 desaturase. This enzyme is essential in turning our good fats into PG1 and PG3 hormones. And what happens to a blocked fat? They get stored as cellulite (nasty adipose tissue). That's what makes your butt all dumpy and gross. Hydrogenated oils. And that's not all. In a relatively healthy individual, it takes 7 weeks for hydrogenated oils to exit the body. And since good fats only last 3 weeks inside of you, quitting the program in under 2 months is hardly enough time to be cleaned out enough. Try this program for the length of time I recommended earlier so that you can see I'm right.

That's also why it takes consistent daily supplementation to replace essential fats and why I say it's at least 21 to 49 days for all the positive changes to be realized by some folk on this program. You're toxic folks! Face it! So if you get a little bloated, experience a little exhaustion or have a headache or two, you know why. The toxins have entered your bloodstream on their way out of the body.

No matter what, do not take any drugs to alter this process. Aspirin, acetaminophen and other anti-inflammatory drugs (like ibuprofen) will pose further problems. These drugs are beneficial only for a short time because they block the negative workings of the PG2 group. However, they also interfere with the PG1 and PG3's. This is why you will burn fat for a little while using those "ECA" stacks but then almost over night, it all stops. What could you do to clear out toxins and hydrogenated oils from your body a little faster? Start incorporating olive oils into your diet. Cook with it and pour it on your green vegetables. Omega 9 fats are great for cleansing the liver.

LEMMONS OIL

All of your other essential fats can be gathered by incorporating 2 egg yolks, a tablespoon or two of Lemmon's Oil, olive oil, real butter and 2 tablespoons of raw cream a day. That's about 30 to 40 grams of very HEALTHY fat. Fat that makes you lean and mean, not fat like a cat! I used to recommend a product that was fairly close to what we need but I use my own blend of oils these days. I do not trust anyone else to make them anymore. I am truly tired of the light colored blends which claim they are something they aren't. My oil is a unique blend of several different fatty acid sources. It meets the demands set forth in this chapter and is not only richer, but thicker, tastier and more nourishing than any other oil you know. It is also fresher by leaps and bounds too. That's right.

You can forget about using oil that is 6 to 12 month old ever again (and that's what they are despite the manufacturer's claim). You haven't lived until you have used an oil freshly pressed just 7 days before you receive it. This oil is Lemmon's Oil. Why did I make my own oil? Well, as each year passed that I was recommending another product, I asked myself why I hadn't done it long time ago. The quality of the blend seemed to dwindle, it tasted more and more stale and the delivery time became far too unpredictable each passing month.

The customer service and the people who ran the company were nothing but a bunch of clowns. Bitter? Yes. Those people raped me and they are raping the public. Tired of being at someone else's mercy, I had all I could take so I put together something BETTER than whatever you are currently using because I felt it HAD TO be done. I couldn't go another month without proper essential fatty acid nourishment and many women I have had as clients weren't tolerating it any longer either.

When we first met, she was severely depleted of her fats. And trust me, you only know what you are missing when you start using a good oil then stop taking it. So, what I did was contact the most reputable natural oil company in North America and explained my situation. Seems my complaints with the previous manufacturer were more than common knowledge in the industry. We moved forward and the result is Lemmon's Oil, which contains only Omega-flo unrefined certified organic oils including:

High Lignan Flax Seed, Sunflower Seed, Safflower Seed, Pumpkin Seed, Borage Seed, Sesame Seed, Almond, Wheat Germ several other wonderful ingredients. The wheat germ oil is used as a source of octacosanol (500 mg of wheat germ oil provides 1000 mcg of octacosanol) and rice bran oil for gamma oryzonol (which contains ferulic acid). Both of these oils have shown positive results in increasing glycogen storage and assisting in effective carbohydrate metabolism (with just 2 grams per 100 pounds of body weight a day).

My oil is high in natural antioxidants, FIBER, blood cleansing and emulsifying ingredients.

When I say it is THICKER, TASTIER, more nourishing and FRESHER than any other oil available, you really aren't going to fully appreciate it until you try some. It truly is the most complete source of essential fatty acids I know of anywhere. This product is the highest source of usable Omega 3 oils available because of the specific mixture and ratios. What we have here is a unique blend that falls into the most natural balance of nearly 50% Omega 3's, only 10% but all healthy saturated fat sources, and just above 20% of both omega 6's and 9's. The dark brown and greenish color of "Lemmon's Oil" displays its flora/vegetation origins.

A far cry from the pale colors the competition offers. If you use this oil and this oil alone, no other oil is necessary in the human diet... Because nothing else compares and you won't pay for expensive glass either. Lemmon's Oil is manufactured with an exclusive low temperature pressing (86 to 99 degrees F, 30 to 37 degrees C) and the processing and packaging (HDPE) is performed in complete exclusion of light, oxygen and reactive metals to maintain the life of the Omega Fatty Acid nutrients. There are no additives, no preservatives, no bleaching agents and no hexane extraction involved in its production. No trans fatty or hydrogenated fatty acids are found in Lemmon's Oil either.

Only certified organic seeds and completely unrefined oils that were not genetically modified are used in MY oil. We use Lemmon's Oil as a condiment on meats and vegetables after cooking them or on my salads and cottage cheese. Sometimes I even have a tablespoon by itself. The taste is a wonderful mix of buttery, nutty, and tangy flavors and it's really smooth going down! Adopt this oil as a regular part of your nutrition plan and you will never go astray again. Vitamins are like a good football team. You need a full team of vitamins on the field every time the ball is in play.

The ball is your life. Sometimes we keep other vitamins from the roster on the bench, watching those on the field, waiting their turn. Each member of your team knows what to do when the time comes and each player has a different job from the others. A good team doesn't bully it's own players nor feed off other members. Each works with its teammate's strengths without depleting itself because vitamins look out for each other. All nutrients are meant to work together this way, and none really stand alone, no matter how important you think they are.

If one vitamin is missing, or if one is in too high of a dosage, then somehow, some way, some where, it disrupts the team. This is what weakens your support structure. Minerals are different from vitamins because they are more like having fans in the stadium. Without fans, there really isn't any support for your team. In other words, there is no motivation for the vitamins to work their hardest without minerals. While some of the minerals are more visible and exciting than the others and may appear to be more important, kind of like cheerleaders, without even just one row of fans sitting in the stands, you can easily tell that something is missing.

The support will not be there like it used to be, and it will show. Even if you do not know what it is for sure that is missing at first, something is definitely not right, and it could cost you the game. What pulls the team together, what pulls the best of all teams together, is coaches. You and I both know that a team without direction gets nowhere. Well, fats are the coaches, trainers and administration that normally go uncredited for pulling the vitamin team together and gathering the fan support of the minerals for a winning effort.

The fans love them for what they do, the team needs them to digest and assimilate their orders correctly, so without having a good foundation of coaches, everything falls apart. You NEED fats. Especially essential fats.... And Lemmon's Oil provides ALL of them.... And if you are interested in trying Lemmon's Oil, if you haven't already, it comes in a 16 oz bottle that yields 32 servings of 120 calories each (these calories DO count in your overall caloric intakes but these fats DO NOT make you fat) and we will be glad to make some fresh for you.

When your muscles do not have enough glycogen which is made from carbohydrates, your endurance is shot, you get fatigued and not only will performance drop, your progress will not exist. How can you assure glycogen is spared? Having enough essential fatty acids available at all times. Follow this rule and in no time at all you will become a physical specimen to behold....

Certainly glandular products which are made from animal organs that strengthen our own have been popular but they too work best when combined with essential fatty acids. For more, visit: www.glandularcomplex.com

SUPPLEMENTS, VITAMINS
AND MINERALS

I remember my first bottle of amino acids like it was yesterday. I bought them for $20 from a guy named Robb Lee in Newton Falls, Ohio where I grew up. He now owns a great restaurant there. These amino acids (protein pills) were made by Beverly International and smelled of pure ammonia. The highest of quality you will find anywhere. I thought I was taking something practically illegal and assumed it was going to make me a muscled bodybuilder overnight just by taking those stinky horse pills. Nothing happened though. I took the entire bottle in a month, 12 or 16 of them a day I think, and yet NOTHING HAPPENED.

I didn't realize I was supposed to start lifting weights to build the muscle. I hadn't a clue. That's the same attitude most people have. Pop a pill, the world becomes a better place. Supplements are supposed to assist you by being an 'extra' boost to your current plan. If the plan is not complete, it can only boost you so much. True for anything you try. If you take a fat burner that boosts your metabolism by 10%, it isn't going to show results if everything else you do continues to reduce the metabolism by 30% now is it? The aminos I first took only served to feed my malnourished body instead of helping it grow muscles. They couldn't possibly help to build even a little muscle. I wasn't eating enough nor lifting weight to substantiate my body to grow.

Six months later, after I was weight training regularly, the next products I tried were mega packs from the local health store. They had a deal where you bought two bags or bottles and they gave you another one free. These at least made a difference because they were my first source of real nutrition (I didn't eat very well).

I was taking like 8 packs a day, 10 capsules of amino acids before, during and after my training too. I wasn't sure what worked, the training or the pills but after a while, I noticed something stimulated my metabolism enough that I began eating more food and more often. Up to the point of eating more, I was getting muscular but wasn't putting on much weight. The next summer, I tried my first protein powder. I replaced fast food with protein powder. Again, I didn't get anywhere all week using it. In fact, I lost muscle that week.

Everyone in this industry wants to sell you treated powdered milk, fake sugars that cause disease, hydrogenated oils that interfere with healing and hormones, synthetic vitamins the body doesn't recognize, filtered and flavored minerals that are useless and pro hormones that the pros wouldn't even bother with. Everyone claims they sell only the best and they wouldn't tell a lie. Well, that's the smoke they are blowing up your skirt. As Willie Wonka once said "We are the dreamers of dreams." This is precisely what they depend upon.

Exactly what role does your health really play in your lifestyle? Are you kidding? It is everything. But if you continue to look after your health for the next ten years as you have looked after it for the past ten years, what can you look forward to in the future? Is the quality of your life really important enough to you that you will make the necessary adjustments? Did you know that in many cases the reasons you cannot meet your goals, burn fat or build muscle nor slow down the aging process due to what's missing from the supplements you take? With the change from glucose as an energy source to using more free fatty acids and stored fat, toxins that were once stored in those fats are now ending up in your bloodstream. Just know, toxins WILL make you feel tired, sick, cranky, hungry, and etc. It's not the food, it's the junk left behind.

You need 'ANTIOXIDANTS' to remove these toxins (and other free radicals and waste products that are in there). No, you won't need a prescription to get them. Antioxidants are nothing more than vitamins and minerals that protect the body from free-radical damage. These toxins are partly to blame for wrinkles, cancer, pain and cramping that occur once cellular damage begins. An optimal antioxidant should be found to contain upwards of 200 I.U. of vitamin E (DE, not DLE. DL signifies synthetic, meaning not natural), 1000 or more mg of vitamin C and bioflavonoids, at least 7500 I.U. of beta carotene, 200 micrograms of selenium, and 15 to 30 mg of zinc. Wait a minute!

The Don Lemmon Multi-Nutrient contains exactly this already! How convenient! Other antioxidants and free radical scavengers like herbs are useful too. We include grape seed extract in ours for this reason but you can never be too careful that some huckster isn't trying to convince you gravel is an antioxidant these days too. Someone is bound to do this sooner or later. I remember when the amount of grape seed extract we use in our formula was $40 a bottle. If it were worth $40 a bottle for exactly what we use, how could we afford to put 100 other nutrients in there for almost half the price? Because anything over priced is NEVER worth getting. It may benefit you, but there is no need to pay that much for it.

Have you been taking other supplements because your joints hurt? I'm not so sure you should be wasting your money on over-priced snake oils, which supposedly prevent cancer as they heal joints. Fishes don't get cancer nor do they get hit by busses. From what I have learned on this subject, it's the plankton that fish eat which protects them from cancer, not their cartilage that most everything on earth is born with. What plankton does is assist minerals into the cells of your tendons. Where are you going to get a ton of plankton on a daily basis anyhow? I certainly believe that other species' cartilage may relieve pain by strengthening your joints because eating chicken cartilage (yes, that's true) does. But cure CANCER? Based upon what? The fact the fish doesn't get cancer? Puh-lease. I would simply double my mineral intake, eat more chicken legs (skinless and not fried or breaded), start having more dark green veggies if not seaweed (which we buy as sushi paper wrap to roll rice with it or we get the weed itself and make soup). If that fails, I would begin taking an extra 500% of the RDA in B-6 and begin supplementing with some RUTIN until the pain subsides.

Rutin is a bioflavoniod from the pulp of citrus fruits that has displayed a role in healing tendons and ligaments in the old and young alike. It is also great for carpal tunnel syndrome. Wait a minute! The Don Lemmon Multi-Nutrient already has 1000% of the RDA in B-6 and contains a great source of rutin!

Who says I haven't covered the bases? All other remedies may fall by the wayside if we keep going at this rate! Even if you do find a product that works in curing disease, taking an antidote after taking a poison only works temporarily in delaying your demise.

Please address the other factors in your lifestyle which you know you should change because supplements do not remove the bad habits which caused the ailment. Getting back to nature, getting back to the basics, ALWAYS works, so let's do that. The other issue I have with supplements are diuretics and water pills. None of them do what the ads claim. While fat is less than 15% water and over 70% fat, and muscles are over 70% water and contain only 6% fat, guess where you'll lose weight from if you use diuretics or water pills?

From wherever the predominance of your water is stored, that's where! Muscle! If you are over 50, growth hormone therapy may help. In very low therapeutic dosages, HGH can help anyone, but in higher dosages, if you are below 40 especially, you are only looking for trouble. You won't see the negative side effects right away, just like with other drugs, that is if the HGH is synthetic, but in 20 years you will. If the form you use requires a needle to inject, look out! You know how a liver donor has to match blood types? Or a kidney needs to come from a relative?

What makes you think that any old source of HGH from some dead person you do not even know, or a cow for that matter, will be tolerated by your body any differently than that? I know most of you will think you need more "stuff" than I recommend, or that I am only trying to sell my own products, but really, you do not need much else. Some other supplements serve a purpose, but usually they are used for limited time and they only work if the product is of the same quality used in clinical studies. More often than not, you can't get that quality. Go buy something you think is supposed to work. You'll see. Especially once your diet becomes secure. That's because if you eat right, nothing except what I have told you about is necessary.

Isn't eating right and taking vitamins good enough then? Sure, eating right does wonders, but food isn't what it used to be. That's why we must adhere to so many rules in order to succeed on food alone. Our soils are depleted year after year from farming, pesticides and hormones leach ever more from what we eat and in most cases, the food is aged by time we have even the freshest of sources ready to consume. Sometimes, it's got at the most a 50th of what food had 50 years ago. No kidding. And what do you think happens when you cook your food? It gets fresher?

Our crops have 98% less of some of the same nutrients in them today as the crops grown in our same U.S. soils using the same testing techniques in 1948. It only takes 10 years of intensive farming to exhaust the minerals in any tract of land. Some of the major farms haven't rested their fields in over 50 years. Besides all that, even the best of vitamins only cover 20% of the necessities your body requires believe it or not. And while taking any old vitamin may help a little if you're really deficient, it is still not going to help you enough unless you also get ALL of your minerals and make sure the nutrients are in proper ratios to one another.

These are the keys along with eating right and getting essential fatty acids that assist your nutrients. Minerals and dosages are what make the difference between any old vitamin and a good product. Vitamins are essential organic compounds. And various amounts of each vitamin participate in the functions of the entire human body. This includes growth, fat loss, mental acuity, dis-ease prevention and energy production. Some vitamins are fat-soluble (meaning they require fat to process) like A, D, E and K. Other vitamins are water-soluble vitamins like the various B-Complexes, C and such (meaning if you are dehydrated, they do not function properly).

Vitamins generally cannot be synthesized by the body unless you deplete yourself of other nutrients to do so. The only time the body makes it's own is when you have crossed that 'danger' zone and are heading into severe malnourishment. The thing is, they cannot be made in adequate amounts under these conditions and this is why they absolutely MUST be supplied by your eating and supplementation habits. These nutrients became publicly known around 1912 when Vitamin A was first isolated.

The others were found one by one up until 1948 or so when B12 was discovered. The term 'vitamin' stems from a reference to the fact these nutrients are 'vital' because the body is fallible without them. Vitamins come mostly from plants and grains except for vitamins B, C and D, which are present in the muscle tissue of animals that consume foods containing them. Considering that only about one-quarter of the people reading this will ever eat correctly each and every day, and since vitamin critics don't adequately recognize deficiencies of the average diet, or what it takes to regain what we have lost, you had better take this seriously.

Each vitamin has specific work to perform inside of you and a deficiency of one vitamin cannot be remedied by consuming more of another. This is another reason why a variety of foods should be consumed on a daily basis. You need a little of every-thing, not too much or too little of anything. Natural vitamins are those occurring in food from animal or plant sources. Synthetic vitamins are usually identical to natural vitamins and if taken with food, the body will recognize them as part of the food. However, a few synthetic vitamins do differ from their natural forms.

Synthetic Vitamin E, called dl-alpha-tocopherol, is a mixture of both left and right handed molecules so to speak, while the natural E alpha-tocopherol is a single molecule form called d-tocopherol. The synthetic product is adjusted so that it pro-vides the same biological activity as the natural form. They do this because it's common knowledge people do not eat as good as they should. They think simply popping pills is all they have to do. "But Doctor, I take a multi-vitamin daily." Really? Does it contain minerals? ALL minerals? Minerals are completely different inorganic (non-carbon containing) nutri-ents that also cannot be formed in the body and must be obtained from the diet.

Minerals are either positively charged (cations) or negatively charged (anions). Cations are derived from metal elements such as calcium, cobalt, chromium, copper, iron, magnesium, man-ganese, molybdenum, potassium, selenium, sodium and zinc. Anions are derived from non-metallic elements such as iodine, sulfur, phosphorus, chlorine, and fluoride (to name a few). Combining anions and cations together synergistically creates mineral salts such as sodium chloride, calcium phosphate and sodium iodide.

And as much as minerals work, play or belong together, vita-mins and minerals are even more dependent of one another than minerals are of each other. You know how some football players are bigger than others? A lineman may be 300 pounds but a quarterback is probably 225? Or a receiver is 185 pounds and a running back might weight 200 pounds? All nutrients follow the same suit. Each 'player' so to speak has a specific daily task that requires a certain amount of support at all times. If a lineman weighed only 200 pounds he would probably get eaten up by the opposing team pretty quick and would be unable to do his job. If a quarterback weighed 185 pounds he would get crushed. If a receiver weighed 300 pounds he would be too large to get his work done.

This is why without a properly formulated multi-nutrient that contains all the vitamins and all the minerals in ratios or weights that allow them to work efficiently, you'll survive, but you won't feel, look or live up to your potential. I used to take a multiple vitamin that contained exactly 100% of the RDA dosages of all the major vitamins. I thought my body needed a little more so I took it twice a day. Well, in time, this proved not to be enough. Why? One, no minerals, and two, like I said, because we require more or less of certain nutrients.

Sure, you may think if you take more than the RDA recommends, the vitamins or minerals will become toxic inside of you but when a person's body is trying to heal, up to 10 times the RDA may be required for a number of different nutrients. The other reason that I stopped using my old vites was that some nutrients can't be taken in 100% of the RDA and expected to benefit you. Sometimes that is way too much. Vitamins are definitely something that should be taken with meals at least twice a day. There are around 20 essential vitamins you need so like I said, simply popping a Vitamin C once in a while or taking any old multi-vitamin or 'once-a-day' caplet is not going to cut it.

I have gone to great lengths in discussing nutrition in this book so far. What I have said may surprise many in the fitness industry as well as the folks who aren't in the industry. And while there are still those of you who refuse to eat right no matter what I say and insist that if you take supplements you read about in an article somewhere that you will still somehow get somewhere, you're entirely incorrect. First of all, you must eat right. Eating bad isn't remedied by popping pills, even if it is my pills. You have to eat right or the body cannot assimilate anything you take. In fact, only once you get your diet together, then and only then should you add supplements.

Next, tell me something. Is the multi-vitamin you are using now a caplet? I suggest that you begin CHEWING your pills if they are caplets. The coating of most pills is typically too hard to digest and your gut cannot break them down. As undesirable as that may seem to chew these things, you might as well get used to it. You will appreciate the fact that the pill doesn't come right back out your tail end anymore either. Oh, sorry. You didn't know that most caplets end up coming through you unused? That's right.

Like I said, the coating is too tough for the enzymes in your belly to break apart. This is why the product I use comes in a soft gel capsule. My product, which I have personally created, is an all natural, patented, and exclusive blend manufactured for me under the strictest of supervision. It was designed using my own research and is based upon clientele feedback and blood tests. The nutrients are in ratios I feel not only enhance the bio-availability of all the other nutrients but increase the uptake of the foods we eat. That's what makes my particular product invaluable! There is literally nothing like it anywhere.

What we have available to us now is a blend of pure science, technology, and essential metabolic function that not only meets, but exceeds my expectations to a point that I have changed my opinion on what I think of the competition. There is no competition. You can literally feel the results taking this product the first day. When was the last time you could say that? The only way I can explain it is that you will feel a sort of mental clarity when you first take them. It's an incredible sensation. You will actually feel rejuvenated without feeling like you have drank a pot of coffee. No jitters cause there's no stimulants. Just proper nutrition. How is that possible?

There are at least 90 of the nearly 100 naturally occurring and essential elements known to man in my product. That's 90% of your nutrition folks. All that's missing are your fats but you get those from Lemmon's Oil. A daily serving of the Official Don Lemmon Multi-Nutrient Formula (these capsules, not horse pills or caplets) provides:

Vitamin A (Beta Carotein Seaweed/Palmitate), 7500 IU: This nutrient is involved in vision, smell, hearing, taste, reproduction, adrenal and thyroid glands, metabolic rate, energy, body temperature, skin, and infections in the throat. It also affects lungs, digestive tract, and wound healing. Yes, it is an Anti-Oxidant (fights the free radicals and toxins which scavenge our cells).

Vitamin C (Calcium Ascorbate), 500 mg: Those deficient in this nutrient bruise easily and their blood vessels are so weak that their gums bleed when brushing them even lightly. Vitamin C is an antioxidant too that stimulates the adrenal glands to manufacture cortisone, which is involved in healing and helps to combat stress. It supports immunity by stimulating the production of white blood cells and fights viral and bacterial infections. Vitamin C normalizes blood pressure, lowers cholesterol, thins the blood, and protects you from atherosclerosis and other forms of heart disease.

Vitamin B1 (Thiamine Mononitrate), 20 mg: B complex vitamins smell because they contain sulfur and nitrogen. If you take oral contraceptives, you are deficient in B1. It is also required for carbohydrate metabolism, along with B2, B3 and B5. B1's responsible for nerve, heart, muscle and digestive tissue health.

Vitamin B2 (Riboflavin), 7 mg: Exercise, pharmaceuticals and consistent sinus problems are signs we require more B2. It is also responsible for converting protein into amino acids. Vitamin G was the original name for riboflavin (B2).

Vitamin B3 (Niacinamide), 50 mg: This is the best form of niacin to take because it doesn't make your face red and flushed. B3 metabolizes bad triglycerides and lowers the risk of cancer.

NOTE: Vitamin B-4 (Adenine) is currently not considered an essential nutrient because it is readily available in grains and cereals. This nutrient must be present in the diet in order for the body to produce adenosine triphosphate (ATP).

Vitamin B5 (d-Calcium Pantothenate), 100 mg: Essential for the synthesis of steroid hormones naturally found in the body including adrenal hormones. In highly stressed situations, more B5 is better than 'just' enough especially if you suffer from allergies. People suffering from rheumatoid arthritis have decreased levels of B5.

Vitamin B6 (Pyrodoxine HLC) 20 mg: B-6 controls temper tantrums, mood swings, PMS, carpal tunnel syndrome and a number of mental disorders, including clinical depression and schizophrenia. B6 depletion has also been connected to immune deficiency, kidney disease, asthma, sickle cell anemia and diabetes.

Biotin 250 mcg: Also known as Vitamin B7 or Vitamin H but it is actually just biotin. However, biotin is essential for metabolizing and controlling protein, fats, carbs, blood sugar, amino, lactic and pyruvic acids. It also aids in the prevention of hair loss so it is good to take a little more. Because it is water-soluble, any excess is excreted through the urine.

Folate (Folic Acid), 400 mcg: Folate is B8 which is Folic Acid B9 which kind of is Folacin or B11 that is yet another form of folic acid too. This nutrient is essential for red blood cell division and immunity.

Alcoholics, pregnant women, people who eat fast foods and the elderly all benefit from this vitamin.

Vitamin B10 aka PABA (Para Amino Benzoic Acid), 30 mg:
This nutrient is for stress and relaxes you without putting you to sleep. PABA aids healthy bacteria, the formation of red blood cells, protects against the sun, and returns prematurely gray hair to its natural color. It is depleted during times of constipation.

Vitamin B12 (Cyanacobalamin), 400 mcg: B-12 is important in healing ligament and disc problems, energy, surgical recovery, anemia, cancer, insomnia, vary forms of depression and stress. But B12 also requires iodine and manganese to process. Laxatives, alcohol, aspirin, antibiotics, diuretics, antacids, caffeine, cooking and being not eating meat all cause us to be malnourished of B12.

They say B12 in the form of methylcobalamin is more absorbable but I am not convinced of this.

NOTE: Vitamin B13 (Orotic acid) is primarily used for the metabolization of folic acid and vitamin B12. It is found in root vegetables and is good for multiple sclerosis and liver-related complications, which leads to premature aging. However, the FDA does not consider it vital for human beings and it is banned from dietary supplements as it is suspected of being carcinogenic.

Vitamin B15 (Pangamic Acid) is also not included as the body only needs it if you are a serious alcoholic or someone with degenerative liver problems that only your physician can diagnose. They may refer to it as the 'hangover' helper.

Vitamin B16 (Amygdalin) is also sometimes known as laetrile or B17 is a nutritional compound of two sugar molecules, (benzaldehyde and cyanide). It is used in an unaccepted form of cancer treatment. This B vitamin is the only one that is not found in brewer's yeast. Despite being found abundantly in fruits and green veggies, due to divided medical opinions, it is not included in this particular supplement.

Choline (Bitartrate), 450 mg: This partner in the B-Complex family works well with essential fatty acids. It improves short-term memory in normal, senile and people in the beginning stages of Alzheimer's Disease. Certain regions of the brain are easily depleted of acetylcholine especially. Diet doesn't boost the level of choline in the brain at all, and without it, most other nutrients cannot reach the brain either.

Inositol, 200 mg: Another B-Complex family member, inositol promotes alpha adrenergic activity which benefits the heart's coronary vessels, clearing cholesterol and burning body fat.

Look, you may feel nothing is missing from 'your' diet and supplements aren't 'essential' but do the math. B-Complexes are quite important. People are recommended to take B-complex vitamins for their allergies, anxiety, acne, adrenal support, arthritis, bursitis, bowel disorders, bruising, cramps, cardio ailments, depression, dermatitis, diabetes, epilepsy and even more woes all the time by dieticians, nutritionists and physicians for a reason. Do B12 'shots' ring a bell? You're depleted.

Vitamin D (Cholecalciferol), 300 IU: Fungus on the feet? Stinky bowel? You're deficient. Vitamin D detoxifies, prevents PMS and breaks down carbohydrates. Many elderly people are deficient in this vitamin, probably due to a lack of sunlight, but more likely due to dietary depletion. Crohn's disease, epilepsy, high blood pressure, kidney disease, liver disease, osteoporosis, and skin ailments are prevalent in vegetarians and those who do not get their fair share of the Big D.

Vitamin E (tocopherol blend), 200 IU: Vitamin E delays many effects of aging, prevents fibrocystic breast disease, edema (fluid retention), is essential in blood clots, scar tissue, burns, headaches, and should always be taken with proper amounts of selenium and Vitamin C. Without enough Vitamin E you can forget about Vitamin A doing it's thing.

NOTE: Vitamin F is a pet term for essential fatty acids like those in Lemmon's Oil. Also note, Vitamins B18 through B-gazillion and Vitamins I, J, L, etc aren't anything to concern ourselves with so I won't be covering them here...

Vitamin K (Phytonadione), 50 mcg: Antibiotics deplete the body of vitamin K. Ever taken an anti-biotic? Did you know it could take YEARS to replace what those drugs deplete? Vitamin K is found in dark green vegetables.

Bioflavinoids (Rutin, Quercitin), 500 mg: While technically not vitamins, 50 different bioflavinoids are found in the pulp of citrus fruits, in pine bark and even grape seeds. They act as antioxidants and are natural tendon and ligament healers that are also dandy anti-inflammatory agents.

Vitamin "P" as they were first known are not essential but if you have aches and pains in your joints, you're going to love us for including them.

Boron (Chelate),10 mg: This mineral is required for the maintenance of bone and normalizing blood levels of estrogen and testosterone. In fact, within a week ladies, you will lose less than half the calcium, a third less magnesium and twenty five percent less phosphorus through your urine than you are used to just by taking this supplement.

Calcium (Citrate/ Chelate), 500 mg: If you are deficient, the thyroid gland fails as the body begins absorbing it from the intestines and bones. You don't want that. And you know those canker sores that develop on the inside of your mouth? They are related to a calcium deficiency too. Canker sores are a form of the herpes virus. Once you have it, you have it forever but if you keep your calcium levels up…

The virus won't manifest canker sores. And keep in mind, calcium deposits are not caused from having too much calcium in the diet but from a lack of what is needed to process it… That's other mincrals and B-complex vitamins!

Chloride (Potassium Chloride), 340 mg: Potassium chloride helps acidify tissues in people when their joints and bursae sacs ache (bursitis). It activates numerous enzymes and is the basic raw material for our stomachs to make stomach acid (HCl) for protein digestion (pepsin - a protease enzyme).

Chromium (Polynicotinate/Chloride), 300 mcg: This does what they say it does. It helps keep blood sugar levels steady so you can fight off cravings for sugar and carbohydrates while burning fat.

Chromium is a mineral that dieters seem to get a little obsessed over but you do not need more chromium in your diet as much as you need all the other minerals. If you insist on taking chromium, use 300 mcg of chromium poly-NICOTINATE (GTF) not picolinate for every 100 pounds of lean mass you carry.

Copper (Gluconate), 2 mg: Many times PMS, candida albicans, and even anemia disappears once a woman overcomes her copper deficiencies. Men, this nutrient is wonderful for the prostate.

Iodine (Kelp/Potassium Iodine), 150 mcg: Iodine is required if like certain people, you have recurrent sinus infections. This stems from an over active thyroid using up your iodine. Iodine will also adjust vaginal discharge.

Iron (Chelate), 4 mg: Symptoms of iron deficiency include listlessness, fatigue, heart palpitations, reduced cognition, memory deficits, sore tongue, angular stomatitis, dysphagia, and hypochromic microcytic anemia. Do you know anyone who chews ice? It is a disorder more commonly known as pagophagia. It stems from iron deficiency anemia. They probably have other cravings for red meats and even some non-food items. Do you or they also chew ink pens and fingernails? You need minerals. That's all. It goes away within the first few days of supplementation. If you are told that iron causes heart attacks, your source is misinformed. The iron we chose to use helps build red blood cells to carry oxygen throughout your body to shuttle the other nutrients to cells for energy and recuperation.

Magnesium (Citrate/Chelate), 450 mg: This nutrient is essential for calcium and potassium assimilation, contributes to proper nerve and muscle impulses and assists in the correction of nervousness, muscle weakness, heart palpitations, light headiness, diarrhea, most hormonal issues.

Fluoride from tap water and toothpaste, refined sugar and corn syrup and artificial sweeteners will deplete you of magnesium in a heartbeat. Magnesium carbonate, chloride and oxide are inorganic forms and are less absorbable than the chelated citrate we use.

Manganese (Gluconate), 10 mg: No, this isn't magnesium listed twice. This nutrient helps the thyroid gland produce hormones, speeds the metabolism function and without it Vitamin C and the B-complexes cannot do their jobs.

Molybdenum (Chelate), 75 mcg: It has been claimed that molybdenum influences the susceptibility to esophageal cancer. Studies suggest that cancer patients are deficient in molybdenum.

Phosphorous (di Calcium Phosphate), 100 mg: A phosphorus deficiency leads to not only osteoarthritis, but kidney stones, urinary tract and tartar on your teeth.

Selenium (l-Selenomethionine), 200 mcg: Also very helpful in preventing herpes outbreaks, preventing cellular mutation, cancers and if you are in treatment for AIDS, try taking 2,000 mcg of selenium daily

Vanadium (Vanadyl Sulfate), 150 mcg: Vanadium improves insulin action, inhibits formation of cholesterol in blood vessels and in the nervous system and improves the mineralization of bones and teeth. Vanadyl Sulfate is a tool used by athletes to store extra glycogen, or sugar, inside the muscle for a more pumped look which could also contribute to greater strength (the extra glycogen, not the pump). Problem is, that doesn't work. The key word is EXTRA.

Vanadyl doesn't help one bit with what the body can already handle on its own in storing carbs really. If you're already full of intra-muscular carbohydrates, then and only then will the body accept any assistance. But if you're full, you're FULL. You can get all the Vanadyl you need from my multi-nutrient and 100 other nutrients at a greatly reduced price than buying Vanadyl alone anytime.

Zinc (Gluconate/Sulfate), 30 mg: Zinc helps with sexual function, mood stability, immunity and prevents body odor.

Grape Seed Extract (95% standardized OPC), 25 mg: OPC's are very powerful bioflavonoids that are assimilated into our body tissues and strengthen the blood within hours!

Essential Amino Acid Blend, 100 mg: Amino Acids are the "building blocks" of the human body. Besides doing all of the above, plus building cells, repairing tissue, forming antibodies, combating bacteria, viruses, being a part of the enzyme and hormonal systems, building RNA and DNA, carrying oxygen throughout the body filled with vitamins and minerals, what don't they do? There are eight amino acids considered essential because they cannot be manufactured by the body and for the sake of better nutrition, here they are. It's not a lot, but it's plenty to do what we need them to. Assist the other nutrients.

Dimethylglycime (DMG), 25 mg: This is another amino acid that specifically stimulates T-cell production, thus its job is to maintain the immune system.

Polyfloramin, 100 mcg: What the heck is this? It is the trade-marked name given to the phytogenic extracts used exclusively in T. J. Clark Mineral products. It is basically all that is good taken from their exclusive blend of plant source trace minerals.

How do you like that? That's a lot of stuff isn't it? Well, it's all of your major vitamins, minerals, plus more B-Complex 'stress' vitamins Anti-Oxidants and trace minerals than any other product like this. Did you like that I have also included essential amino acids? There is just enough in there to make sure all the other nutrients have 'back up' to do their jobs!

I also used to take extra trace minerals on top of my regular vitamin and mineral supplementation, but not any more. Can you believe on top of it all, this particular formula contains a full day's serving of colloidal minerals? Like I said, no corners cut, nothing left out, all bases are covered! That's over 120 total nutrients using this system! Aren't you excited?

When we got our first batch I felt like dancing, hitting the gym, going for a run, something... And I truly believe that the key to it all was the extra trace (colloidal) minerals we threw in. Why colloidal minerals though? What makes them so special? We know the major minerals build bone, muscle tissue, and support the nervous system. Colloidal minerals promote the utilization of major minerals like calcium (boron) in saving your bones, the breakdown of sugar and carbohydrates (chromium), the building of red blood cells (cobalt), stronger teeth (with natural fluoride), enhancing thyroid function (iodine), fighting cancer (manganese), protein synthesis (molybdenum), fighting free radicals (selenium) and they even have antibiotic capabilities which help heal wounds by producing white blood cells (zinc). And this is just a short list.

The following colloidal minerals are found in Don Lemmon's Multi Nutrient Formula: Antimony, Arsenic, Aluminum, Barium, Beryllium, Bismuth, Boron, Bromine, Cadmium, Carbon, Cerium, Cesium, Chromium, Cobalt, Dysprosium, Erbium, Europium, Fluorine, Gadolinium, Gallium, Germanium, Gold, Hafnium, Holmium, Hydrogen, Iridium, Iron, Lanthanum, Lithium, Lutctium, Neodymium, Nickel, Niobium, Osmium, Oxygen, Palladium, Platinum, Praseodymium, Rhenium, Rhodium, Rubidium, Ruthenium, Samarium, Scandium, Silicon, Silver, Strontium, Tantalum, Tellurium, Terbium, Thallium, Thorium, Tin, Titanium, Tungsten, Vanadium, Ytterbium, Yttrium, and Zirconium.

Still don't think vitamins and minerals go together? Look at a bottle of Anti-Oxidants sometime. You will not only notice that these products consist of both vitamins and minerals but my product supplies more nutrients than anyone else's does. The fact remains, a proper supplement is made up of both vitamins AND minerals, not just one or the other.

And if I can squeeze 120 nutrients in every single capsule, who do those other companies think they are fooling with their for- mulations? They only hold back what they offer you in their products so they can force you to feel the need to buy more than one product! It's simple marketing! They are cutting you short on purpose! Notice anything else in Don Lemmon's Multi-Nutrient that you have been buying separately and paying an arm and a leg for up until now? Well, don't do it anymore! People that are taking lithium for depression can find it here for pennies! Chromium? It's in there! Colloidal silver? We got it! Vanadium for carbohydrate metabolism? That is in there too! Amazing isn't it? No need to buy 50 different products every month. Take just this one multi-nutrient combined with Lemmon's Oil and you're all set.

Still think minerals are unnecessary? Got tartar on your teeth? That's a bonafide phosphorus deficiency. Take this product for a month and see if it helps or not. It will. And if you are a sweater, you are acidic. So not only do you need more minerals because you perspire more than most, but you need more minerals to stop the sweating, or at least control it. It's just another common mineral deficiency. No, Gatorade doesn't even come close to lending a hand (I have to laugh at that one)!

Even Dr Linus Pauling, the 2 time Nobel Prize winner in medicine and the King of the Vitamin C movement said "Every sickness, every disease, every ailment known to man can be traced to a mineral deficiency." Top that. Do you suffer from neuralgias, psychoses, eczema, poor sleep, lupus, herpes, hot flashes, obesity or any of the above? Maybe you don't now, but later in life as you begin to age due to malnourishment you might. ALL these disorders are commonly associated with stress but it's really due to poor metabolism of B vitamins, not the actual lack of B-vitamins. It's a lack of the minerals needed to use the complexes.

You bet, in fact, niacin and thiamin are totally useless without both minerals AND essential fatty acids in your system. So again, don't forget your Lemmon's Oil! Go team! Vitamins, minerals, trace nutrients, anti-oxidants, b-complexes, plus amino and essential fatty acids are the things that combine with your foodstuffs to create and maintain all your enzymes, cells, hormones, tissues, metabolic needs and even slows down aging. There isn't a function you can name that isn't protein, fat, vitamin or mineral dependent.

Many of the companies you recognize that sell vitamins and minerals dilute theirs with water, juices, sugars and other synthetic ingredients. This weakens your product. You can be certain that this particular product is free from artificial flavors, sweeteners, colors, corn, gluten, yeast, wheat, dairy, soy, preservatives or pesticides. This program is the Rolls Royce of nutrition AND health and you need your supplementation to complete it. You do DESERVE a Rolls Royce don't you?

If you are ready for a full month supply of Don Lemmon's Multi-Nutrient (180 capsules) for $30 U.S., which includes shipping, simply drop me an email or visit <u>perfectvitamin.com</u> today! Lemmon's Oil is only $20.00 a bottle shipping included. Drop me an email or visit <u>www.lemmonsoil.com</u> and let us know. Also let us know I told you that if you buy one, the second bottles are half price!

Carbohydrates, proteins, and fats. Vitamin, minerals, and essential fatty acids. Getting sleep and making sure what goes in one end comes out the other. Certainly herbs are turning heads these days as well. They contain phytochemicals store bought foods do not have which heal us. For more, visit: www.ultimate-herbalformula.com

THE IMPORTANCE OF WATER

If you feel that you are retaining water even though you drink water all day long, or if you rarely go to the bathroom then you probably SIP water all day and don't realize you have to CHUG it. If that's what you do and you're still bloating and not peeing, you had better rush to a doctor. That's not right. Since the odds are more likely that you are dehydrated, I suggest doubling your water intake and adding more fiber to the diet. Besides everything else we have discussed, by far the most important thing the human body requires next to air is water. Water makes up the largest overall percentage of our physical being (muscles alone are comprised of over 2/3 H_2O).

It regulates numerous functions which otherwise slow down without it like maintaining the elasticity of your skin, eliminating wrinkles, lubricating joints, balancing blood volume, controlling the ability to attack viruses, getting rid of constipation, urinary tract issues and generally everything else from sleeping to thinking. With this in mind, you should try to drink a gallon of filtered, purified or distilled water for every 100 pounds you weigh each and every day in order to provide yourself with a proper level of hydration.

This amount of fluid will suffice in eliminating the urge to drink coffee, tea, fat producing juices, sodas and other liquids that you really don't need. If you do drink one of these other liquids, don't worry yourself over it, just be sure to have an extra equal amount of fresh clean water to wash it down. You need to go pee-pee as often as possible the first couple of weeks. By then, your bladder will adjust to the new routine. This is important to know because every time you pee the body excretes toxins and flushes your fat right down the toilet!

So, drink enough at all times to keep your urine clear. Letting it turn yellow is a sure sign of a set back. Water should be drank upon waking, 15 minutes after each meal, between each meal, before, after, and during workouts, before bed and then again at all other times you feel thirsty. That is approximately a dozen minimum daily servings. A gallon of water has 128 ounces. Divided by 12 that is only 10 ounces of water 12 times a day for each gallon you are to complete by day's end.

If you are required a gallon and a half, that would be 15 ounces 12 times a day. For 2 gallons, have 20 ounces at a time. I weigh around 200 pounds but am pretty active and I currently live in the desert (Las Vegas, Nevada) so I personally keep a 24-ounce cup full of water by my side or on my desk at all times. You should drink water throughout the day, even if you wake up in the middle of the night. Especially if you wake up with muck (dry) mouth. Drinking water at night or in the morning before getting up through a straw (still laying down) is a good thing because your valves stay open while lying down and that allows for a faster quenching of all your tissues.

As we grow older, our thirst mechanism is less efficient. We sometimes have to remind ourselves to drink. So always have that glass, cup, jug or bottle handy and full of fresh water to keep yourself reminded. The glasses of water you drink between meals should be cold if possible. If you are obese, make that water not just with ice in them but actually ICE COLD. The internal cooling effect the ice initiates inside of you will speed the metabolism up (to warm you) and you'll burn more calories. When I say ice water, I do not mean you should be sitting around sucking or eating cubes. If you have this habit, it could stem from what is known as pagophagia.

It is a disorder that is commonly associated with iron deficiency anemia. You probably have other cravings for food and some non-food items too. Do you also chew your ink pens and finger-nails? This is relevant in 50% of such patients with a mineral deficiency. That's all it is. Luckily over 70 different minerals that your body requires is in my Multi-Nutrient Formula.

If you do not like the taste of water, in time, you will, but for now, add some fresh lemon or apple cider vinegar to it (especially if you have a cold as this kills bad bacteria). I get my apple cider vinegar from Omega Nutrition. It's made the old fashioned way which leaves all the vitamins, minerals, amino acids, pectin, fiber, healthy bacteria and enzymes intact. Be certain you only have this cold water with cider or lemon juice in it BETWEEN meals because the acids could destroy your digestive enzymes. They boost your enzymes if you use them between, but during, no way. And make sure you get the cider from Omega. Regular old store bought isn't good enough.

As far as the water drank with or after meals, it should be room temperature and SIPPED, not chugged or gulped, if drank at all, during the meal. Having 4 to 8 ounces sipped at a meal is fine, that doesn't hurt. But drinking a lot of water to 'wash' your food down mid meal is not a good idea. If you do not pay attention to these things, you will have trouble digesting your foods, let alone flushing nitrogenous waste, toxins, body fat and even poo-poo out on a 'regular' basis. Just remember, if you dehydrate, kidney function is tweaked, waste products accumulate, and the body's sole reaction is to retain all the water it has left. You will bloat and until you get enough water back in the system, your engine cannot become healthy again. The liver will certainly try anyhow (stressing itself out) attempting to flush out the excess waste on it's own.

As a result, fat burning is shut down and you become fatigued, bloated, aggravated at the drop of a dime and did I mention migraines? Oh, you already get them? I wonder why... Next, I suggest getting a home water filtration product of some sort. You may get by without it, and you may think your tap water is alright, but in most cases, fish would die if left alone in the average glass or tank of plain old tap water. Trust me, if a gold fish can't survive in tap water, it can't be good for you either.

Don't stop there. I want you to get a good shower filter too. You are what you absorb and everything you are trying to avoid by drinking only purified water will still get absorbed (through your skin) while bathing anyhow. Hey, you are washing in tap water. You don't have to drink it to absorb the chemicals in it so be careful. Tap water contains chlorine, which destroys the healthy bacteria in your gut, and that is what makes illness difficult to deal with. This is also why I said that when you buy your water, you should shoot for distilled water. I do not trust what is in spring water nor what is in most grocery store bought drinking water either. Many brands are nothing more than filtered tap water, which is sometimes fine, but it's not boiled of all impurities like distilled.

Here you thought you knew all there was to know about water. So, let's recap. If you weigh 100 pounds, drink one full gallon a day (128 ounces). If you weigh 125 pounds, have one and one quarter gallon a day (160 ounces). If you weigh 150 pounds, have one and one half gallon (192 ounces) and 175 pounds a day requires one and three quarters gallon (224 ounces). If you weigh 200 pounds, that's 2 gallons a day and so on and so on. Yes, if you weigh 300 pounds, I expect you to drink 3 gallons of water NOT SODA between waking up and going back to sleep each day. This is hardly a lot to ask!

ARTIFICIAL SWEETENERS

I don't care how bland you feel your food is, there is nothing wrong with the way natural foods taste. Thinking you need artificial flavoring on everything is a sure sign of how chemically dependent you've become. I have had many clients who abused their intake of artificial sweeteners to a point they needed medical attention. Do you really want it to go that far? One woman I used to know in particular ate 120 packets of artificial sweeteners a day. Yeah, 120. And her withdrawal symptoms were horrifying. Things like nutra-sweet, aspartame, sucralose, splenda and saccharine are not natural foodstuffs. They are chemicals.

They are drugs. Drugs, that when their temperature exceeds room temperature, like inside the body or a cup of coffee, converts these wood alcohols into formaldehyde and formic acid. You know what that is. Formic acid is the same poison found in insects like fire ants and scorpions. Sure, not as much, but enough to cause metabolic acidosis and methanol toxicity that gives innocent victims symptoms of multiple sclerosis. I have been given reports of people suddenly beginning ['to']tremble, becoming blurry eyed and even hearing bells in their ears after drinking diet soda.

If you suffer from any disease symptoms such as spasms, joint or organ pains, numbness in your limbs, cramps in your muscles, sudden dizziness, headaches, depression, anxiety, slurred speech, or memory loss and you are using chemical sweeteners, then you need to stop whether you think it is related or not. The memory loss is due to the aspartic acid used to make these sweeteners. It goes past the blood brain barrier and deteriorates your neurons eventually causing seizures.

The phenylalanine used to make these sweeteners is mutated so it depletes serotonin, causes manic depression, panic attacks, rage and violence in otherwise calm, cool and collected individuals. I realize the sugar industry has added artificial sweeteners to our foods but relabeled those foods as healthier alternatives but if they aren't harmful to begin with, how can you label something as healthier or SAFER? Something is either healthy and safe or it isn't. If you say SAFER, are you implying that before, it wasn't safe enough? Sounds fishy to me. I honestly feel nothing can be done to stop the distribution of these chemicals in our foods but we can refuse to buy or eat anything that contains them.

That's a great place to start. I personally stopped drinking decaf coffee once I found out the industry uses bleaches and formaldehyde to remove the caffeine. I am not a caffeine junky, but I do like my occasional coffee and once I began to avoid the formaldehyde, man, my health did a complete turn around. I couldn't figure out why, even though it was decaf, I still got the jitters. Have you ever drank a cup of decaf and suffered a little 'night' blindness in the middle of the afternoon? That was the formaldehyde poisoning your retina.

The methanol in your artificial sweeteners converts to formaldehyde. Formaldehyde is just like cyanide and arsenic. It attacks nerve endings, changes body chemistry and causes neurological disorders even when taking the smallest amounts. I used to tell people to just limit their intake but now that I know and have experienced the difference myself, I demand you stop using them immediately. If for no other reason, stop using artificial sweeteners because they are also part of the reason you crave carbohydrates. Do you remember what happens to extra carbs? It becomes hard to reach body fat. What do carbs mixed with chemicals become? Cellulite.

And any formaldehyde that hasn't damaged you yet, will, because it is stored in your fat cells, particularly those in the hip and thigh areas. Yummy. Do you like carrying around grotesque, jello-looking, bouncing, cellulite? This is also another reason why when you start to lose fat on this program that you feel so nasty and crabby. Your fat cells are dumping out all those stored chemicals for excretion. Live with it because sooner or later, you won't have that choice unless you rid yourself of this gunk as soon as possible.

And trust me, the manufacturers of these poisons know how awful for you they are. Their funding/lobbying of the American Diabetes Association, American Dietetic Association, Congress and even the American medical associations is nothing more than blood money. So, what's the solution for a sweet tooth? Besides trying to just get used to the natural flavors of food, there is always stevia. Stevia is a natural herb and food sweetener, which also helps in the metabolism of sugar as opposed to tricking your body into thinking it too is a carbohydrate. That's what these artificial sweeteners do. They trick your body into thinking it's getting sugar so you'll still suffer from insulin woes on top of everything else.

From now on, if it says "sugar free" "no sugar added" or "dietetic" on the food label, check for what chemicals it contains before buying it! Even if it says "fat free" or "nonfat" still read the label. Companies like EAS and Met-rx are poisoning you with artificial sweeteners, hydrogenated oils and cheap ingredients. You do not even realize it nor do they care. Most people may think modern medicine has all the answers but the latest medical research is released daily that proves the marketing hype to sell artificial sweeteners wrong. You know it, I know and it's time everyone else knows it. Spread the word. You'll thank me one day.

Friends don't let friends drink diet soda, use protein powders or eat foods that contain artificial sweeteners. I had a decaf coffee recently that I was told happened to be a naturally caffeine free blend. I was also told the creamer in the container was real cream, not artificial. I didn't have 3 sips before my speech slurred, my vision blurred and my head pounded. It took a 3 hour nap to recover. All chemicals are poisons. Mix them with hydrogenated oils and you're killing yourself.

When I say I do not know a single athlete, model or body-builder that has more than one meal replacement shake a day, I mean it. In fact, I had a rather well known spokes model for one best selling protein powder brands on the market announce on my radio show that most of the before and after pictures her former company used were fakes. Another mutual friend has endorsed a particular line found in grocery stores for the past 5 years says she cannot use the stuff at all. It gives her hives! What's in that crap? Crap.

GOURMET RECIPES

Barbequed Chicken: Gather 2 pounds boned and skinned chicken breast halves, 1 small chopped onion, 1 small can tomato paste, 1 large minced garlic clove, 2 tablespoons sugar free Worcester sauce, 2 tablespoons apple cider vinegar, 1/4 cup unsweetened pickle relish, 1/4 cup unsweetened red or white wine, 1 teaspoon sea salt and 1 teaspoon dry mustard. Mix all your ingredients together and pour them over the chicken breasts in a crock-pot. Cook at low heat until tender.

Chicken Kabobs: Gather 2 cups chicken broth, 2 tablespoons vinegar, 1 pound boned and skinned chicken breast halves and one third each medium red, green and yellow peppers cut into one inch pieces. In a small saucepan, mix the broth and vinegar over medium heat until it smoothes out. If desired, add fresh parsley and rosemary. Cook it until the mixture boils and thickens, stirring it constantly. Thread the chicken and peppers alternately on 4 long skewers. When done, place the kabobs on a lightly oiled grill over medium-hot coals. Grill uncovered for 15 minutes or at least until chicken is no longer pink. Turn and brush it often with your broth.

China Chicken: Gather 2 tablespoons soy sauce, 2 teaspoon chicken flavored low-sodium bouillon, half teaspoon ground ginger, 1 pound boneless, skinless chicken breasts cut into strips, 2 chopped garlic cloves, one cup bean sprouts, 1 red pepper cut in strips, one half pound fresh string beans, 8 ounces fresh sliced mushrooms, 1 small onion cut in strips and 8 ounces sliced water chestnuts. Combine a half cup of water with the soy sauce, bouillon, and ginger in a bowl. Mix it well and set aside. Next, coat a large skillet with nonstick spray, add your chicken and garlic. Stir-fry it for 3 minutes over medium-high heat. Once done, remove the chicken and stir-fry your veggies until they are tender but crisp. When ready, re-add the chicken back along with the water chestnuts and bouillon mixture. Cook the mix for just a few more minutes or until thickened.

Orange Roughy: Round up 1 cup sliced onions, 2 tablespoons olive oil, 2 cloves minced garlic, 1 sweet yellow pepper cut into rings, 1 can

Spanish-style stewed tomatoes, 2 ounce jalapeno peppers, 1 pound orange roughy or any other lean white fish fillets, a dash of garlic powder and a dash of ground red pepper. Sauté the oil, onion and garlic for 5 minutes or until tender in a large nonstick skillet over medium heat. This is when you will add the sweet yellow pepper and tomatoes and cook over medium-high heat for 3 more minutes. Next, add your fish, garlic powder and red pepper. Cover, reduce heat, and simmer for 5 minutes at which point you will turn the fish over and cover and simmer 5 more minutes or until fish flakes when tested with a fork. Finally, transfer fish to serving plates with your sauce spooned over it.

Salmon Vera Cruz: Gather four 4 ounce salmon fillets, one half cup fresh lime juice, 1 tablespoon dried onion, a 12 ounce can of tomatoes, and 1 teaspoon dried parsley. Place the fish in shallow dish, combine remaining ingredients and pour them on top of fish. Bake uncovered at 400 degrees for 15 to 20 minutes.

Spicy Sirloin Steak: Round up 1 pound sirloin steak, 1 tablespoon chili powder, 1 teaspoon ground cumin, 3 large minced garlic cloves, 2 teaspoons unsweetened Worcestershire sauce, 1 teaspoon sea salt, one half teaspoon freshly ground black pepper, a quarter teaspoon allspice, a quarter teaspoon ground cloves and 1 tablespoon extra virgin olive oil. Begin by trimming any and all fat from the steak and cutting it into three pieces. Mash the other ingredients together into a paste and rub it all over the meat. Marinate in a zip lock plastic bag for 30 minutes in your fridge while you prepare the grill. Next, cook the steaks over hot coals until done to your liking. Serve with salad.

You might want to get a grill to cook with. My out door grill isn't big and only cost us $30. We also have an electric one than plugs in the wall and sits on the counter too.

Sirloin Steak with Mushrooms: Gather 2 pounds boneless sirloin steak, 1 pound portabella mushrooms, 12 ounces regular mushrooms, 2 cloves of minced garlic, 3 large shallots, one fourth cup butter, 2 scallions, 8 ounces cup balsamic vinegar and 4 tablespoon soy sauce.

Cut the steak into 4 equal pieces seasoned with sea salt and black pepper. Combine shallots, garlic, half the vinegar and 1 tablespoon soy sauce in a zip lock bag. Shake it up, add the steaks and let sit for 3 hours. Cut your portabella mushrooms in half, then cut all the regular mushrooms into four pieces each and chop shallots and scallions into halves. In a skillet melt half of the butter and add half of the shallots.

Warm over medium heat for 1 minute before adding portabellas and seasoning with salt and pepper. Simmer for 15 minutes then transfer to a bowl but keep it warm. Now, repeat the process with the other mushrooms except this time reduce the cooking time to 10 minutes. In a separate bowl, mix 3 tablespoons of soy sauce and half the balsamic vinegar. Add this to your mushrooms and boil them for 3 minutes or until the liquid is slightly thickened. This is when you'll add the scallions. Now is also the time to preheat the grill. Cook the steaks about 5 minutes per side and serve with your mushrooms.

Teriyaki Steak: Get 2 pounds of flank steak, 2 tablespoons chopped red onion, 2 tablespoons organic canola oil, 2 tablespoons organic apple cider vinegar, 2 cloves of minced garlic, and 1 teaspoon freshly ground unsweetened ginger. Cut the steak into serving pieces and trim off all visible and excess marbled fat. When done, place it in a shallow baking dish coated with oil. Combine the remaining ingredients in a bowl and mix them to pour over the steaks and then let them sit in the refrigerator for 2 hours covered. Preheat your grill 20 minutes before removing the marinade. Place steaks on the heated grill and cook until done. That's about 5 minutes per side. Brush them with remaining marinade periodically throughout. Serve over steamed summer veggies.

Creamy Potato Mushroom Soup: Gather 2 soy bacon strips, 2 cups of chopped mushrooms, one half cup chopped shallots, 4 cups cubed Yukon gold or baking potatoes, 1 can nonfat chicken broth, 2 cups non-fat milk, 2 tablespoons sherry, one half teaspoon sea salt and a quarter teaspoon ground pepper. Add mushrooms and shallots with bacon to the pan and sauté for 5 minutes or until the mushrooms are soft. When done, remove from pan and set aside. Put the potatoes and broth in the pan and simmer until the potatoes are tender (about 10 to 15 minutes). Immediately transfer the potato mixture to a food processor and process until smooth then return it to the pan. Next, add the milk, mushroom mix, sherry, sea salt, and pepper and cook over low heat for 10 more minutes or until it's thoroughly heated. Top with crumbled soy bacon if you like.

Low-Fat Wild Rice: Gather 2 cups of either nonfat vegetable or chicken broth, 1 cup water, one half cup wild rice, one half cup white rice, 12 ounces sliced fresh mushrooms, 1 minced clove of garlic, a half teaspoon of sea salt, 1 pinch saffron, 8 ounces chopped green onions, 4 ounces chopped fresh parsley, 2 teaspoons lemon juice, and a couple parsley sprigs. Bring your broth and water to a boil over medium heat in a medium saucepan. When it boils, add the wild rice to simmer, covered. After 20 minutes, add your white rice, mushrooms, garlic, sea salt, and saffron. Simmer 20 more minutes or until rice is tender and most of the liquid is absorbed. That's when you'll stir in the green onions and parsley and let stand for 10 minutes. Just before serving, sprinkle the lemon juice and add the sprigs of parsley. Serve with black beans.

If you go to a restaurant and like the meal you have ordered, do not be afraid to ask about speaking to the cook or chef. On one hand, you might discover the meal wasn't prepared properly after all but the idea is to possibly weasel the recipe out of them. Don't be shy, most of the time they are more than happy to let you in on their secrets.

Sun Dried Tomatoes And Capers: Get together 4 sun dried tomatoes, 3 freshly peeled and chopped seedless tomatoes, 3 tablespoons minced red onion, 3 tablespoons of capers, 3 minced garlic cloves, 2 tablespoons balsamic vinegar, 1 tablespoon fresh chopped basil, 1 tablespoon fresh chopped oregano, 1 teaspoon freshly ground black pepper, sea salt to taste and grated nonfat Parmesan or Romano cheeses. Place the sun-dried tomatoes in a small bowl with 1 cup of boiling water until it cools when you will drain and finely chop them. Preheat the oven to 350 degrees. Combine all other ingredients in a bowl and set aside for an hour at room temperature topped with the tomatoes. Sprinkle with your cheese if desired and add to pasta.

Santa Fe Pasta: Round up 8 ounces sliced green onion, 2 minced cloves of garlic, one and a half diced medium red and green bell pep-pers, a half teaspoon of sea salt, one half teaspoon chili powder, black pepper to taste, 1 dash of cayenne pepper, 12 ounces evaporated nonfat milk, 1 tablespoon cornstarch, 8 ounces fresh cilantro leaves, and a half pound of pasta measured dry, but cooked. Cook the green onion and garlic in large skillet over medium heat for a couple minutes. Add the bell peppers, sea salt, chili powder, black and cayenne peppers then cook for 5 minutes more. Mix remaining ingredients then add to the pan and cook over medium heat until it's all slightly thickened, stirring as necessary. Take pan off stove and serve over pasta when ready.

I have a few additional ideas that you might want to replace in the fridge. You never know what is in a cream or a sauce that allows it to stay bottled for months on end....

Healthy Mayonnaise: Mix 1 tablespoon lemon juice, 1 whole egg, 1 tablespoon tarragon vinegar, 1 tablespoon unsweetened Worcestershire sauce, 1 teaspoon sea salt, 1 teaspoon mustard, and 3 tablespoons Lemmon's Oil in a blender for 20 seconds. Then slowly add more oil. Amount of oil varies depending desired consistency. The mix shall thicken once chilled. Keep refrigerated.

Bleu Cheese Dressing: Mix one whole egg, 2 tablespoon tarragon vinegar, 1 tablespoon unsweetened Worcestershire sauce, 1 teaspoon sea salt, and 3 tablespoons Lemmon's Oil. Put the mix in a blender for 20 seconds. Add 4 ounces of bleu cheese and blend until it all thick-ens. Slowly add a little more oil depending upon your desired thick-ness. Keep refrigerated.

Milkshakes: Another easy way to liven things up, substitute entire meals or to add a couple of snacks if necessary is by making. milkshakes. But meal replacements are normally nothing more than hydrogenated coconut oil, bleached corn syrup, powdered milk and if you are lucky, they add some multi-vitamins to it too. Hidden behind a health food marketing campaign, I admit, some of them taste great and shakes add variety and convenience to your diet, especially if you are on the go like many of us are, but you aren't supposed to live off of the chemicals they put in them. Steer clear of anything claiming to be a meal replacement.

I mentioned using a blender, but believe it or not, some people do not KNOW HOW to actually use a blender. You can't just dump stuff inside of one and turn it on! Some things will stick to the sides and others will jump right back out at you if you do.

1. Make sure the blender is clean first and big enough for all your soon-to-be blended goodies. The bottom of the pitcher twists off, remove it. Clean that too, along with all the glass parts, inside and out, then screw it back on with the ringlet back in place and TIGHT too.

2. You can now add your liquids, creams, diced fruits, and non-sticky solid items. Other items may include sweeteners like sugar-free cocoa, syrup, molasses or honey and nonfat dairy products like milk, ice creams, yogurts, and acidophilus. Other 'milks' could be rice, coconut, or soy. Diced fruits and berries are good if they are unsweetened, fresh, frozen or chilled.

I mix oats, nonfat milk, cinnamon and frozen blueberries almost daily. Once inside the blender you can put on the lid and start it up (on low at first). Gradually increase the speed until it looks like a whirlpool in the center. If it doesn't blend that well, add a little water.

3. While it's spinning, add the dry ingredients but watch closely so that they do not stick to the sides before blending. If necessary, use a spoon to dislodge anything that does stick (without digging too low and losing the spoon in the cutter at the bottom). After you add the dry ingredients, if it appears too thin, add ice cubes. This thickens it back up and keeps the shake chilled. That's why I use frozen blueberries. I also add wheat germ, oat bran, or other whole grains to my oats too.

Just a few tablespoons will do. Another option: Broccoli! It adds a nutty taste to the shake! If I use protein powders, I use pure pulverized whey protein powder with little to no carbs and add ice cubes made from cream. Make sure the label of your powder says it contains the amino acid Tryptophan. No protein mix is good without it. All natural protein sources contain each of the essentials and if it is devoid of tryptophan, it is not a natural source. Ladies, keep in mind, protein DOES NOT mean you're using a weight gainer. It's 'just' protein. You need it. But you don't need it with carbs.

4. Shut everything off once it is blended, unplug and enjoy! Soak your blender in hot water when you are finished so it is easier to clean! Nothing worse than a crusty blender!

I know these milkshakes sound cool, but do not put protein powders in with your milk and carbs.

DIFFERENCES BETWEEN PROGRAMS

This program is based upon what works with, as opposed to against, the human body's natural mechanisms. After working with thousands of folks ranging from the dis-eased, obese and anorexic to clients with close to 300 pounds of lean muscular body mass, I am certain I have found what REALLY WORKS. Not only that, but I know how to keep it working. Without the same hands on experience such as I have put into this, without the same passion I have put into this product, ANY-BODY ELSE'S theory, while possibly an educated guess, is still only A GUESS.

That is why many of my competitors have failed you. No passion. Not as much experience as you'd think. Most of them are nothing more than mouthpieces and spokespeople. I have worked with and spoke with most of the leaders in the body-building and fitness industry. I have literally gathered information from all around the globe and it has always come down to being the same old story. Most people achieve their goals by accident. Hard work and perseverance are taken into consideration, but if you ask people what works, they are still looking for it. It's amazing.

This chapter was written to address the readers who feel they know something I do not. I never claimed to know everything there is to know but what I do know has left quite a few people more than envious. So this goes out to those of you wanting to say I am wrong in one way or another even though you're not sure why. Hey, I made sure all the facts are right here for you to review. I could go on for hours giving you more to go on and yet no matter how much sense I make, there are always going to be those of you saying they already 'know' or believe something else other than I do.

I am not sure how that makes me incorrect. Well, do your own research. Examine a few basic medical texts. Tell me another time who is right on the money. Or at least send me a copy of your own book while you're at it. Besides, if 'everybody knows' this or that, why are so many people still out of shape while following 'this' or 'that' then? On this program, I have seen muscle weight increase from 180 to 240 pounds. I have seen others go from 150 to 210 pounds. I have seen the diabetic decrease their insulin dosages. I have seen the hypoglycemic lead a normal life.

I have seen the elderly tone up. I have seen chubby kids become fit young men and women. All it took was changing their eating habits. What you have learned getting this far through the book should explain why what you have been doing up until now may or may not "work" after all. You should also now have a pretty sound idea why some of what you are doing will NEVER work. But then again, I too realize there remains a small percentage of you reading this book simply out of curiosity whom continue to feel that unless you follow a lower fat diet, the Zone diet, the Atkins diet, food combining, 40-30-30 nutrition, the Protein Power plan or a vegetarian routine, you can't succeed. I must have failed in saving you.

Most diet plans have just enough truth to them and contain enough commonly known facts to make them appear credible or at least difficult to totally discredit. That's what sucks you in only to fail again. And just in case you believe that you need to study your blood type at a school of higher learning to assure results, I suggest having your blood tested immediately. Certainly. And keep the results. Do this so you can see for yourself and show everyone you know how much nonsense you used to believe. Have the plasma, erthrocytes, leucocytes and platelets all examined.

That's all four major constituents of your blood. Just ask for a "CBC" test. Go back and have it all done again in 6 weeks too. See if it mattered one bit what your blood type was when you started after all. You owe yourself that much. Remember, you can actually follow any of the competitive diet plans using the food separation advice I have given you in the 12 Food Groups. Try me for 6 weeks. You might finally get somewhere. I hope you were able to grasp at least that much already. And no, I haven't forgotten about those of you who are Body for Life cultists nor the high fat dieters in our congregation today (I am joking about the religious over tone)…

I haven't forgotten any of you. I certainly haven't forgotten the fitness pros and doctors you revere either. Just understand, only a fourth of medical schools OFFER nutrition to their students and only 1 in 4 of those actually TAKE the course. We're not talking about requiring the credit hours to get into medical school or offering it as a secondary degree here. We are talking about these people that you put your faith into only having at the most 12 credit hours, and sometimes LESS in nutritional education. And you are learning more today than most fitness professionals have in all the years they have worked in or around the industry. I am not condemning the medical or fitness fields but I do insist you take control of things on your own for a change.

Your health practitioner may like to remind you that they know best because they are physicians or your trainer might think they know best too but that's often only to bully you from asking questions. If being in the medical profession was all it took to be so smart, why aren't ALL doctors in agreement? Because they are in different branches of their field? Ok, why then do so many doctors in the same fields of medicine disagree? Because they all know so very little about nutrition.

They weren't taught it in school and they do not practice it at home. Titles mean nothing. It's TOO EASY for them to simply brush off someone telling the truth when it saves their butts for having misguided you all the while anyhow. Even worse, dieticians and nutritionists these days are being pumped out ['of']schools like robots or puppets on assembly lines too. They are taught their ABC's about certain areas of their field then set free to dispense their newfound knowledge upon the world. Sadly enough, it's painstakingly obvious so few of these people conduct actual research outside of what is required of them to graduate. They are parrots for their cult. Why do I say that?

I can't help but question why so many nutritionists, dieticians and other food industry professionals are so sickly looking, fat, and out of shape if they know something more than what I am telling you. It's hard to find a registered dietician or a certified nutritionist who look their part. If you find one, that's the exception, not the rule. Trainers too are limited in knowledge as well because for some reason, their certifications only cover the basics as set forth by the AMA (American Medical Association) and they usually learn all they are required in an 8 hour week-end course taken at their gyms.

Back to square one. I hope you realize that just because someone has a certification or a degree in this or that, it doesn't make them qualified to dispense advice on these subjects I have covered. I cringe at the thought some trainers are employed at all. And, guess what else? If you believe what you read in the magazines or hear in the news about your eating, you've been misled again. By who? By those doctors, nutritionists and trainers who've now listened to those handling the marketing of your favorite diet or fitness products.

These people only get away with it because they know you're desperate enough to believe and willing to try anything to see results! All I am saying is that the fitness industry is hardly run by professionals with any real qualifications. It is run by people trying to make a buck or two off of people like you, hoping you believe everything you are marketed. So if you believe Bill Phillips or Metrx are 100% honest, you probably believe Britney Spears sings her own songs in concert or the Backstreet

Boys created their own dance moves. It doesn't matter if someone has a best seller either. They will come and go. Pet Rocks were best sellers at one time too my friend.

Yeah, yeah, surprise, surprise, you thought the people in the white lab coats, the ones you read about in the magazines or saw on late night TV were the prophets of our times and had all your answers. Wake up. They are for the most part borderline clueless, lying through their teeth to cover their tracks or just trying to sell you something. You've all been misled. I put this system together to serve myself. I didn't write it for you or anyone else in the beginning. In fact, I hid what I knew for a long time.

It wasn't until I saw what the industry was doing to us each passing generation that I started giving my advice away. I didn't even charge a dime for it either until I realized I wouldn't be able to put solid effort into actually serving people unless turned it into something I could do full time. I have come a long way since then but I do not flaunt flashy cars, brag of having several homes, or wearing expensive jewelry. You're more likely to catch me in a t-shirt, blue jeans, baseball hat and tennis shoes at a $4.99 buffet than you are seeing me pay $50 for a fancy meal dressed up somewhere needing reservations.

In fact, I give my lectures in jeans and a t-shirt most of the time. I am no different and no better than anyone else, unless of course, you are counting my desire, passion and sincerity towards what I do. I love to meet new people and am not greedy about setting consultation fees. I will often hook up with out-of-town clients for the price of a buffet, so do not think for a second I am wearing different pants than you do.

Since this all began, my clientele has now extended and grown to thousands of people. Each one of you have wonderful stories to tell. Every walk of life from soap opera stars, television personalities, Playboy Playmates and yes, everyday people like ourselves who do all sorts of things from all across the globe have been on this program. I have seen people experience a tremendous amount of fat loss on the exact same program used by those that were looking to gain weight. And I mean obscene amounts of weight gain like going from 160 to 225 in six months (while not gaining even a single ounce of fat) on the same routine another person used to go from 450 "oh my God, that's fat" pounds down to 225 pounds and looking like they were never obese to begin with.

I know, you want to know more about the celebrities I work with. What did they do? The same program. Well why don't I list more of them then? Catch 22. From 1996 to 2000 I had the winners of virtually every single professional female fitness event in the World come film for my workout videos, on my program or have some sort on involvement with me. Mr. America Lee Apperson was in one video, Danny Weigand, a USA Champion, was in another. I could go on and on. You've probably seen my site already.

But why didn't I use more famous people if I work with celebrities? Hmmm. Many current and former clients are rock stars, politicians, super models, actors, professional athletes, fitness stars and body-builders and are not listed or discussed because for one, most are under endorsement contracts that do not allow them to 'advocate' me and two, because others like their privacy. No one wants the world to know they put on a few pounds, you know ? And since I do not pay the others for their testimonials, it only makes sense they look else-where for funding their careers.

Maybe one day I will consider sponsoring some of my clients but it is not within my budget to pay the latest home run king or academy award-winning director for their public support. I cannot compete with soft drink or athletic wear manufacturers. Don't ask me about the bigger named supplement companies either. Body For Life or any of the other 'transformation' programs you can count on one hand are designed entirely on getting you to buy $300 a month worth of products from the ringleaders of the system. Look at whomever is sponsoring the contests. It's someone selling a product line. Never fails. Sure, some say you do not 'have' to use 'their' products but you better if you expect to get recognized!

I remember when Body For Life used to require receipts for your supplement purchases to even enter. Most of the time, if there is that sort of hype surrounding a specific supplement line, like Met-rx, that means they are trying to make big money, sure, but that's also a clue that there is something they aren't telling us too. Meaning it's not what we think it is. Why would you need so much hype if you had the magic product? Wouldn't word spread on it's own? Why would you need to promise someone fame if they succeed? Because that's what it is all about.

People want recognized and told they are as good or better than the next guy. Know right now that you already are. Besides, if Met-Rx were really a 'metabolic prescription' which is what the medical term 'met-rx' stands for, why not call it that? Because it isn't one. And so you know, it costs most companies only 10 cents to fill a packet full of meal replacement powder while they turn around and sell it for $4 each at the health food store. I remember when it used to be that if you bought health food, it may have been expensive, you at least got what you paid for. Go out and read whatever you like. Learn. Explore.

After reading this book, you will spot the hidden agendas of others right off the bat. I am sincere when I say I am devoted to human health and drug-free physique enhancement (with or without the desire or genetics for bodybuilding, weightlifting, modeling, or athletics). I have put everything I own including my heart and soul into formulating this program and our two prized supplements. This book and those two products supply us with 100% of the essential nutrients science tells us we need just to survive. Nothing more is necessary. I do not care who's program you follow, if you apply at least that much, your routine will work better.

I do not ask you to buy creatine, glutamine, meal replacements, or any other mumbo jumbo from me. In fact, if you do not want to try my products at all, you still need those 100 nutrients. Creatine is not technically part of your food. It is something that exists in your body but it isn't necessarily an important food nutrient. The body makes it's own out of other nutrients that are in the foods that contain it. Ironic, I know. But that's how it is. You see, all those guys taking extra with their food are actually confusing the process and preventing the body from absorbing that and other nutrients.

If you take the creatine between meals, or AFTER a carbohydrate meal and you have over 200 pounds of lean mass, it should work. I do not mean taking it directly after. I mean using it between a carb and a protein meal. So if you are going to have carbs at 8:00 a.m. in the morning and protein at 10:30 a.m. then 9:30 a.m. which is halfway between finishing your last meal. Hypothetically that is 8:30 a.m. Mix the creatine in just a little bit of water, swish it in your mouth, hold it there a few seconds and then finally suck it down. Creatine is most efficiently loaded when taken in the presence of elevated blood sugar levels like after a carb meal.

If you take it with your food, or sugar, that's not going to be enough time for the body to raise that blood sugar. You'll get nowhere. And with or without my supplements, you also need to put what else I have taught you into action just to see for yourself if I am right. Don't listen to anyone else. If I am showing you a side of myself you didn't expect to see, good. Let's get it all out in the open. It isn't a matter of "Why is this guy talking to me like this?" It is more of the question of "Why am I not listening to him yet?" I may not bend on my beliefs but that's because bending is what got you here. It's time for change and being nice hasn't convinced you to do so.

I had the same fears about change as you do at one point. Sure, I have been working with people off and on since 1986, starting off in Ohio where I was born and eventually moving to North and South Carolina then Los Angeles and Las Vegas. But I wasn't always sure of what I was doing either. Even when I was considering a career in orthopedic surgery, I knew that something was missing from the 'wholistic health' portrait the medical world painted.

I wanted to follow a different path. I didn't know what needed changed, but something did. Oh trust me, I have seen, heard, tried and experienced so much since I started weight lifting just to gain a few pounds as a teenager. Back then I wanted to eat right, whatever that meant, but had little guidance. I remember coming home and having bacon, cheese and breaded fish sandwiches before my workouts thinking it was good in providing me protein. The last diet that I remember being on, that really catapulted my quest for the correct eating plan, was a low fat, low carbohydrate diet I was supposed to be on for 4 days followed by a low fat, high carbohydrate diet for 4 more days.

It rotated back and forth between the two alternatives again and again for some reason. What stumped me, after feeling myself go from flat to fat week after week, was why other people would continue to do this to themselves. Fit to fat, fit to fat, blah. Nonsense. I figured this whole low carb thing followed by the high carb loading phase 'had' to have some sort of a happy medium where one could simply be eating right, not yo-yoing around. Couldn't it? Why couldn't it work if you had just 'enough' carbs? Not too little but not too much, 'just' enough…

Something just didn't add up to me still. In fact, my friend Dr. Dave Williams from Las Vegas, Nevada will remember our conversations on what I called dietary 'happy' balances. We agreed it had nothing to do with 'all things' in moderation. No, because people use that term as an excuse to eat cake and candy not essential fats and clean food. I just didn't know back then how to explain it. I only knew how to accomplish it. So like with that last diet I followed, I noticed that if I ate real lean, say mostly tuna and chicken and vegetables during the week, I would definitely get leaner but I also looked 'flat' because of not eating any starchy carbs. My muscles were depleted and empty.

I actually found myself dreaming at night about cheating on my diet in my sleep. I know I wasn't the only one suffering through such a thing but I also knew that I wasn't having these nightmares when my carb intake was higher. I was being starved. So, I evaluated the routine. After 4 days of carbs, I was sick of feeling fat. Instead of having 4 days of low carbohydrate intake followed by 4 days of loading up on carbohydrates, I had a different plan. We decided we would eat high protein and veggies during the work week, then Friday night we would let loose.

I worked and studied during the week. He worked too. Like every other student and 9 to 5'er, I wanted to enjoy myself those 2 days of the week and relax. So that's what we did. As soon as the boss sent us home on Fridays, we ordered pizza. I liked mine low fat vegetarian style. Saturday morning would be our breakfast buffet (of eggs, sausage, bacon, and cottage cheese) at the local diner. Saturday afternoon was the steak house buffet (carbs mostly like rice, pasta, potatoes and salad). And Saturday evenings we split a case of beer. Hey, just being honest. I drank beer. I also said I knew I needed a change and here I am evaluating exactly what that was...

Sunday's lunch (without fail) was always six 99-cent double cheese burgers (I would throw out the buns) but all the other meals were typical snacks like yogurt, chicken breasts, fish, etc. It didn't take a genius to determine if you eat this much on weekends, you must be REALLY depleted from what you weren't eating during the rest of the week! My body was craving things and I was literally sucking them down. By the end of each weekend, no matter how well I ate, and I did eat clean most of the time, I still felt bloated.

It wasn't just that I was loading up on both carbohydrates and protein, my metabolism had slowed during the week and 48 hours wasn't enough time to speed it back up. I knew I was eating good food, despite the beer, but I was still depleting myself and feeling like I fattened up all over again. And I was getting sick from colds or flus too it seemed every single month. Enough was enough. I stopped. By the end of the next six month period of simply eating the same foods and separating them from one another, like having carbs at only a couple meals a day instead of 14 of them over a weekend, I went from 195 puffy pounds to 215 lean pounds.

I hadn't changed my overall calorie intake at all either. I had found a happy medium instead. I quit the 2000 calories a day for 5 days followed by 6000 calories a day for 2 days and added it all up to average 3200 calories a day. That's what I ate. 3200 calories a day. Those depletion diets always said you should eat your carbs without fat or protein if you want them to load properly without bloating yet they had you eating carbs, fats and proteins together to gain weight. I didn't understand how one was supposed to lean you, but the other fattened you. And why would you want that?

I realized that I was feeling better eating carbs alone at some meals and only proteins and fats at others, but not so good when I cheated and had ate all three together, but how could I have better results than ever before with so little effort? I wondered why someone else hadn't recognized this before. I became a walking testimony that the stomach has no means by which to digest commercially processed foods or separate poorly combined foods. I was living proof and that's all there was to it. Wow, it was like yesterday. Then again…

Sometimes I feel like I just woke up one day training athletes and celebrities in Vegas and California and yet it's actually been so long ago that I figured all of this out. What began as a courtesy of putting friends and patients on eating plans that I myself had been following has turned into something so much more. Food Separation was at first just something that I felt was natural. I was in fantastic shape year round, my health was returning from where I really didn't want it to be and I was only exercising twice a week. So I knew I was on to something. Results are based upon nutritional habits, not my efforts in the gym.

Still, for a while there, many unanswered questions like 'why does it work' were being asked by my clients and I wanted to be able to provide them answers. They do not teach nutrition in medical school folks. So I was on my own if I wanted solutions or answers. This is what led to my research, studying, reading, and eventually writing this very book. If I hadn't wanted you to succeed in life as much as I have, I wouldn't have stepped down from the medical field and we wouldn't have Don Lemmon's Know How. Right now, all I ask is that you willingly climb out of the hole you dug for yourself and get in gear.

If that bothers you, it still isn't me that you are mad at. I understand you may have dealt with a few fitness industry nightmares in the past and are afraid of failing again. I feel for you but I am not allowing you to use what's happened to you in the past as a crutch any longer. You can and I do expect you to depend upon me. So co-operate with me here and I will co-operate with you. I know this is all very new to you too like it is to everyone else reading my book for the first time and you are simply trying to sort it all out in your head before deciding to start. Problem is, trying to apply logic to what you know so little about wastes all the time you could have spent trying something new. By the time you got around to knowing more about what I suggest, you could already have washboard abs if you'll only start today. It took me YEARS to straighten all this out and you're just wasting away whether we agree or not.

No one wants to feel like they didn't 'know' something. But how could you of known something unless you were taught it or discovered it? That's what I am here for. Let's promise one another not to quit just because where we disagree isn't on whether what I do works, but whether you understand WHY it works. We all know how to operate a car but you won't catch many of us designing one anytime soon. All I know is that if I take care of my car, sometimes see a mechanic and stick a key in the ignition, my vehicle will last me a long time and run properly.

One sure fire reason our approach works is not only because proper mixtures of food complements your digestive system so well but it's this fact that ALLOWS you to eat more often and have more food. More food means more nourishment! It's not a ticket to over eat, but your old 1000 calorie a day diets are now a thing of the past with us. In fact, many women start this program at 1800 calories a day and men start somewhere near 3000 calories a day. Can you imagine? Eating like royalty while experiencing results you never before dreamed possible! By looking before you leap, thinking a little before putting something in your mouth from now on, you can do exactly that! NO MATTER THE PROGRAM!

I am sure whatever program it was you were on last probably did in fact work for a while. If you toy with your calories a bit, eat a little cleaner or better than you did before, maybe stopped having fat with carbs or vice versa and started to exercise a little more, most all programs do work for a while. Anything can show minimal results and it's those results that pull us in thinking that it's the only thing that will work for you. Despite those minimal results that had you swearing by your program for however long you were on it, you're still here today for a reason and I have a handful of questions to ask.

1) When did that last diet finally QUIT working for you?
2) Why all of a sudden did it fail at all?
3) Did that diet leave you with unattractive loose fitting skin or more than 10 pounds of fat left to lose?
4) How do you get yourself out of such a rut?
5) Can you see your abdominal muscles at all?
6) Was anything you followed even close to being a practical program you could follow forever?
7) Were their lifestyle limitations?
8) What kind of shape was the author in?
9) Did the author have plastic surgery or take drugs?
10) Are you paying more for your supplements than you are for food each month?

You now know by alternating carbohydrate and fat/protein meals (which yes, somewhat lowers your overall intake of carbohydrates and is a combination of both low fat vegetarian dieting and low carbohydrate meat eating), you can work out the glitches of any program you have ever tried before or are currently following. If you have been eating a low-fat diet, separate your proteins and carbohydrates and add a couple low carbohydrate meals to your daily schedule. If you have been eating a low carbohydrate diet, no problem!

Have some more fibrous greens and add a couple low fat 'no meat' meals to your daily schedule. If you have been mixing proteins, fats and carbohydrates on a diet that leaves you eating in a zone of 30% proteins, 30% fats and 40% carbohydrates, all you have to do is to place the carbohydrates you eat in meals separate from the proteins and fats. If you are on a physique transformation plan that recommends eating 40/40/20 at all your meals, again, begin food separation and try pouring all those powdered meal replacements down the drain. That alone will make all the difference.

Vegetarians, do not eat tofu with starches and add some organic cottage cheese or farm fresh eggs to your program. It's not so much to ask. You wouldn't be here either if what you were doing was fulfilling you. Don't get mad at me for saying it. You know it's true. This book is nothing more than a compilation put together by myself reflecting my years of effort as a collection of information from different readings, findings, communications, etc, etc, and personal notes based upon the needs and results obtained or required from thousands of people, but no single reference is afforded a lengthy quotation that already hasn't been credited. I have come to believe either you KNOW HOW to do what you do or you DO NOT.

If you go to a doctor, a nutritionist, a dietician, a fitness expert , health food store employee or a personal trainer, let alone a supposedly professional athlete and they have a pot belly, saggy skin, double chins, blotchy flesh or look like they haven't touched a weight in decades, do you really think they have any clue whatsoever about what sort of advice you need to make yourself fit?

They aren't fooling me one bit.

THE BODY IS A DRUG

Women usually think if they exercise, all their fat somehow will automatically disappear. Instead, they get bigger. Why? Nutrition. Not exercise. Nutrition. They build muscle but do not burn fat. They haven't started eating right yet. All you need to do to look better than you do today, tightening up the belly, the saggy underarm or get rid of some of that extra caboose you have following your tail, is burn your subcutaneous levels of fat (that is what's under the skin) and that's done through diet. It's all just fat but because you have less muscle under it than you could or should, you'll never look quite right unless you build up a bit.

I guarantee, if your arms are flabby, your tummy has extra folds or your booty needs it's own zip code that within 30 days you will be wearing t-shirts, smaller pants and looking in the mirror again with confidence. It never fails. That is, if you're willing to accept the second phase of the project. E-X-E-R-C-I-S-E. I want you to know right now, if you have skimmed the previous chapters and have not applied the diet to your lifestyle yet, then you are not ready to apply this exercise schedule either. I understand you may be very anxious and think because I look the way I do that exercise must be the secret, but it's not.

The first route to looking better is diet. Training comes. If you don't understand why, reread the 200 pages of the book again. If you ignore the diet and try to jump into the training program without eating right, you are going to fail or at best, remain exactly as you were when you started. No questions asked. Without proper nutrition you are running blind into an iron clad cell made of barbells. It does not matter your sex, age, weight or condition. You need some sort of exercise. You may not be as strong as you like, nor desire to become super duper strong.

That doesn't matter. You still need to keep your muscles, joints and bones fit to prevent getting arthritis, start building muscle, burning fat and getting more or at least maintaining mobility in your old age. Kids begin running and jumping almost from the moment they learn to walk. Supervised training in the gym is safer than unsupervised outdoor activity. Obviously, activity is vital to continued development or they wouldn't become restless when they aren't up doing something. They run around and climb trees like monkeys but rarely seem to get hurt. They fight and wrestle until they pass out because they do not know any better to quit before they tire.

Yet somehow, it makes them stronger and physically fit. With strict supervision, and great patience on your part they build their co-ordination, common sense and motor skills up, training should begin at any age they take interest in it. Power lifting on the other hand should be reserved until after high school, if ever pursued at all, but all other aspects of what you learn today can be applied to the young as well as the old. I am interested in getting kids started on a good exercise and nutrition plan early in life and continuing to educate them because I want more kids growing up healthy with habits they can bestow upon their own children.

Educated correctly, we can eliminate the concern they will turn to steroids, get addicted to caffeine or energy stimulants, orthopedic surgery or anything else we only need to experience once to regret forever. Ignore anyone's advice who obviously has used drugs to get where they are. Whether it is a weight loss or a weight gain drug, still a drug. The routines I offer specialize in short cuts to achieve specific goals in reduced periods of time and completely drug-free. This is the first time ever I have made them publicly available.

Pharmaceutical, recreational and illegal drugs close bone epiphysis and halt linear bone growth by the way. So they really do stunt your growth. Steroids are fourth in line to cigarettes, alcohol and marijuana abuse amongst our children in the U.S. and caffeine is number 6. Teenagers are more likely to break a bone or tear a ligament than any other age group here too. I do not know how it is overseas, but I do know other countries aren't as squeaky clean as they pretend. We all have areas to straighten ourselves up in. I almost tried drug once. But I didn't. And that's what makes me a winner no matter what I do.

Even if I am only second best or just able to keep running in the race, I am a winner because I got there honestly. I do not understand how to build a microwave oven but I do know how to make it work. And even so, the first time I tried to microwave a hot dog at age 12, I burnt my food. Over time, with trial and error, I eventually figured things out. On occasion, I turned to someone for help, but I didn't ask for it if I didn't need it. Maybe you think it's too late for you to put any effort into something new or ask someone questions, but you cannot succeed unless you get up and do your share with what you know.

While I have never helped to build a 300 pound bodybuilder drug free, neither has anyone else besides that person himself using drugs and let's be realistic, these type of people are really not role models. They poison their bodies in hopes of earning minimal paychecks for their efforts. I have helped produce bigger and leaner bodies than a comparable cycle of drugs could on many a client. Problem is, just as there are so many NBA athletes over 7 foot tall playing amongst those at 6 and a half foot or even 6 foot tall, none of them made themselves taller to compete.

They made themselves BETTER and worked HARDER with what they were born with to excel against the competition. With work, we can all get BETTER. With shortcuts, we all pay the price later in life. I had a roommate once who came home with the intention of purchasing illegal fat burning drugs. He told me if I was interested in some, he could hook me up too. He didn't tell me he had them already, he just implied he was thinking about it. I told him no thank you because that particular drug tears you apart inside in the process of supposedly helping you look better outside. Later in life, he would be hating it once his organs began to fail. A week later, I found the drugs in the back of our freezer. I was shocked.

At least when I reminded him again about all the dangers, like losing his health and possibly his job (he was a firefighter), he reconsidered. You see, no one who sells them will tell you that some drugs do not show their side effects on you for a good 20 years. It takes that long for the little scratch they make on your organs to become full-out knife wounds. I am going to assume all who are reading this now are currently drug free. Steroids are not magic beans. There is no such thing as magic beans. Do not be mad at me for saying that. It's true. If you think I am lying then why aren't more drug users looking like professional bodybuilders?

Because there is more to this than taking pills or poking your butt with needles, you only have yourself to be upset with if you're a user. Anytime you think to yourself 'How dare he say that?' while reading this book, realize, it isn't me you're troubled with. It's you. You know you can fully support your own decisions. Following a crowd will get you nowhere. What if that crowd is heading the wrong direction? I want two points to come across here. One, no one around you can do any thing for you other than what you can for yourself and two, if you turn to anyone for guidance about MY system, you're crazy. Why wouldn't you turn to ME instead? I have worked with thousands of people over the years. I know what you need. You eat, sleep, live, breath, parent, celebrate, move and are pretty much so much just like anyone else that I have counseled, so please, turn to only me for anything regarding this program.

I am the one who wrote this, no one else has. And yes, I expect more of you than you ever have. But I do this because I know it is in you to be everything you ever wanted to be. You are capable of anything you set your mind to, including the decision to be stubborn. I realize being stubborn is more about having fear than anything else. This is not anything else you have tried before. It's a wake up call. If you are not ready to drop all pre-conceived notions, I am not ready to teach you.

However, since the next section of the program addresses exercise, let's continue on with steroids for a moment. I know some of you do not care but these drugs slowly, over years, cause your kidneys to fail if nothing else. 10 years after you take even just one steroid, you'll see. You'll forget by then you did this to yourself, but after a decade passes and you start getting pains in your mid back below the ribs, you'll now know why. Don't your kidneys malfunction naturally as we age anyhow? Sure, there are diminished glomerular filtration rates, decreased creatine production, a drop in tissue mass and urinary disruptions as we age...

But why head there any faster than necessary? Besides, there is no evidence that this is a natural path we follow as we age. It is a result of our lifestyle habits. I believe it is a route that only the lazy and those who unwittingly mal-nourish themselves travel. That's the reason I often recommend older generations to supplement with creatine their first month on the program. As we age, the body doesn't produce as much creatine and if you eat poorly, things get even worse. Just think about Granny's skinny and yet saggy arms. There's no muscle there. She doesn't eat right nor exercise.

One, you need to build muscle. Two, you need to eat right. Three, you need to exercise. But that's beside the point. If you are taking drugs, think about that urine bag you'll also be carrying with your saggy arms later in life. And do not kid yourself, girls are doing drugs too. If you have an athletic daughter, she, like many young girls, may think steroids will increase her strength and endurance. Longtime steroid users may lose their breasts entirely and can also result in thickened or lengthened vocal cords. Her voice could deepen an entire octave if she isn't careful. If you teach your children or athletes to win at any cost, they may pay the price for the rest of their lives.

INTRODUCTION TO WORKING OUT

You may have attempted an exercise program before and quit. You may have found that there were time constraints and discipline requirements that were interrupted by your current lifestyle and it was just too 'difficult' to maintain everything. You may now be exercising all the time and haven't seen progress since the Berlin wall went down. No matter what your current schedule or physical condition may be, much of what you think is a 'normal' lack of strength, flexibility, range of motion, balance, endurance, dexterity and posture, etc., all have nothing to do with aging, but rather a lack of what you do to prevent it.

You probably understand that you need regular exercise, or maybe you already do, but I am also sure that you don't know what this really means. Even if you are a seasoned pro, you DON'T KNOW. Too many people are spinning their wheels, including those who are at the top of the game. Many do not realize that the same effects of not exercising at all while we age is also what happens to us when we spend our lives exercising INCORRECTLY too. That is why many athletes are falling apart as they age. It's too much. You may want to excel at sports, tone your thighs or even build the confidence just to get out of the house and meet your soul mate.

No matter the reason, you need to start the diet, not take drugs, and you need to start now, not later to get the results you want. Exercise is the same thing you are doing when you take your car out for a drive once a week during the winter. If it just sat there for too long, the wheels would get rusty and the battery would die. Your body isn't much different. Weight lifting is the stimuli needed to start your engines, keep the wheels rolling and the key to a long lasting battery.

Nutrition is the fuel of all systems involved and what the engine requires to function. Weight lifting, 'training' or 'working out' are the same things. Each can be defined as the act of performing a various number of sets of specific repetitious movements using one or several different pieces of equipment. It is accepted that you will use a certain weight or level of resistance that is predetermined before picking up that weight as well. Simple enough. What's that really mean? Well, for example, bench presses are a single exercise and barbell curls are another. Each exercise is selected because it supposedly targets a particular muscle group.

Bench presses are selected to work your chest and barbell curls to work your biceps. Once you select an exercise, you will then determine a weight to use and probably need an idea of how many times you plan to lift it once, twice, three times or more before stopping. As far as how often to weight train, I usually suggest to my clients that they start off with a schedule where they are working out at the most every other day. It doesn't take secret equipment. Just good equipment. It doesn't take secret supplements or drugs. Just basic vitamins, minerals and essential fats along with a good diet. As far as working out 4, 5, 6 or 7 days a week... 3 days a week is sometimes too much. Even for a bodybuilder. Usually 5 workouts every two weeks with 3 of those workouts being harder than the other 2 are plenty.

So, every other session is one you will put your efforts into. I suggest putting enough effort into them that each workout shows a strength gain better than the last attempt. And no matter what, no workout should ever last more than 18 to 20 minutes in length. How much of a strength gain? I had a lady that was around 50 years old come to me back in 1997. Kathy Faix was her name. She was a nervous wreck because she was heavier than ever and had never really worked out before. She was a full time worker, married, and had two grown kids.

Those kids were in college and did I mention her cholesterol was double what it should be? Well, immediately I put her on the same program I would put anyone else on and in no time she went from 180 pounds all the way down to 140 pounds. This might not seem good enough for people wanting to go from 140 to 120, or those looking to gain weight but bear with me. This lady lost so many inches that she began wearing clothing she hadn't worn since she weighed less than 120. She had completely restructured herself using weight training, the diet and very little aerobic exercise.

As people mature, their bones change. Keep that in mind. Your structure is always going to be a little different than it was when you were younger. But this doesn't mean you won't look better than you did when you were younger. Knowing that Kathy had a cholesterol issue and that she was passing middle age, I couldn't start her off using the weights she ended up using. We began with using a 45 pound bar for bench presses, 50 pounds on pull downs and 90 pounds (which she thought was too much).

By the end of 13 weeks, having gradually increased her resistance and diet to accommodate her building bones and strength, we not only ended up having her bench 135 pounds by herself, but doing over 600 pounds on the leg press (you read that right) and performing her own pull-ups using her bodyweight! And her cholesterol dropped hundreds of points in the process! We experienced similar results with an 80 year old retired steel worker that same year and a 30 year old client went from 160 pounds of blah to 200 pounds of athletic looking muscle doing the exact same workout Kathy used. I even had a high school kid that was considered too skinny by most standards drop 6 inches of fat off his waist and put on 35 pounds of muscle in under 9 weeks with us.

Sure, some say teenage kids exist in a naturally higher anabolic environment than what we do as adults, but that's not true. The difference isn't whether we are in our developmental years.

The difference is in the amount of effort you put into your training. One thing that the older big guys do not have that the younger little guys do is the desire to push as hard as they possibly can to reach a goal. It's desire. I think the big guys have simply lost focus after years of effort with nothing to show for it and they just do not try as hard as they used to anymore. They don't want it as much as they think they do I suppose.

This high school kid however really wanted to bust out of his shell and didn't want to be the little guy on the block anymore. I also want to say that if someone is in the gym for more time than we are each session, they are foolishly doing nothing more than maintaining themselves. We trained 20 minutes at a pop, 5 sessions every 2 weeks and that's it. If you are unfamiliar with the specific exercises or machines I mention, get a complimentary training session from your gym and learn the following:

Leg Extensions, Leg Curls, and either Leg Press or Squats for your lower body. Flat Bench or Machine Chest Press and Dumbbell Flyes or Peck Deck for your chest. Overhead Military Press or Side Lateral Raises for your shoulders. Underhand Grip Pull downs and Bent Over Rows for your upper back. Tricep Pushdowns or Overhead Extensions for your triceps and either Machine or Dumbbell Curls for your biceps.

For your stomach, learn either Crunches or how to use a Nautilus Abdominal Machine that has a pad for your chest to push down upon. Trust me, learning just half these one day and the other half a second day is plenty enough to give you a 'pump.'

You'll get a good workout and can switch things around for variety later on down the road. If you do desire more, I have a free web page made to show you how to perform these and several other exercises. Just email me about it if you want to practice them at home instead of wasting time wandering about clueless at a gym.

DO NOT HESITATE IN CONTACTING ME FOR THIS INFO. MOST IMPORTANT TIP OF ALL: No matter the exercise, your head must be up, your hips rotated forward, shoulder blades back, spine up right, elbows stay beside up and behind you, not on you... And exercising less than twice a week is like not exercising at all. I do not care what Mr. Universe tells you. He was LYING.

What you need to know you are about to learn. You may want to discard what you think you know before proceeding. I do not expect you to understand why this simple approach works, I merely expect you to adhere to the recommendations.

I have heard, seen, tried and done it all since I began this game. I have done 2 hour long workouts, 60 minute routines and even 5 minute sessions. My best results came from reverting back to the basics almost every time, so let's begin there.

Mike Coy, construction, Walnut Creek, CA - "This may seem elementary at times or maybe you don't even understand why it works, doesn't matter, read it and do it anyhow. This program works. I have body built, been a pro wrestler, and worked with a lot of different systems over the years. This IS what works."

Kathy Young, Baskin Robbins Corp, Burbank, CA - "I was just able to do 10 straight pull-ups the other day. 3 weeks ago I was only able to perform 2! No one thought it would be possible but now that I have lost 20 pounds of fat, gained 10 pounds of muscle, and I can finally see my abs too."

EXERCISE 101

Before beginning to lift weights, you need a warm-up. You will want to move about a bit, get your juices flowing, squat down, reach over head, bend over, back, twist, turn around, jog in place for a moment. Run like Rocky up a flight of stairs if you like. Take some deep breaths and as soon as you begin to break a sweat or feel your body temperature finally matches room temperature, it's time to take your crack at the exercises. If it is really cold out you may want to warm up with a few minutes of stationary bike riding, jumping jacks or a brisk walk before weight lifting.

Only you know if that is necessary or not. I am not there to judge but always stop the warm-up once you break a sweat. Doing more than this is part of what makes you sore the next day. Believe it or not, the object is not to find out what makes you sore, but what makes you feel not so sore. Being sore isn't a sign of progress. It's a sensation caused by connective tissue damage (cumulative mirco-trauma at a cellular level) and waste that's built up from the training. Things like the amino acid hydroxy-proline becomes present after you train and it irritates your nerve endings.

You do not want this stuff trapped inside your freshly worked muscles as it hampers progress. This is the main reason why you must wait perform an aerobic (cardio) activity after you weight lift, not before. Aerobics get fresh blood into your muscles to begin the healing. That's really all cardio is good for until you've lost most of your fat. If you do much more than that, before you're around 10% body fat for men and 15% for women, you're going to wish you hadn't. Muscle loss anyone? Pick any one of the exercises I have mentioned or select others you know or something from the website.

One per muscle group is all you'll need and then let's begin. As either a beginner or an advanced trainer, one set per exercise is all you normally require, however, if you live in a cold environment, have low blood pressure or are nursing an injury, I am not opposed to doing a little extra something to warm up. You need mentally and physically prepared for the session. But do not waste too much energy on getting ready. Going through the motions with a lighter weight is more than enough. Sneaking something heavy in to lift masked as a warm up will only hold your progress back.

Trust me! I have NEVER met someone needing more than 3 total sets per movement and two of those were always warm ups. Ever. And that holds true only for only one or two of the exercises in the entire workout, not every exercise. The general rule of thumb is to have one warm-up for every 100 pounds of weight you plan to use. Until you can lift something heavier than your bodyweight, even doing only one set per exercise more could be too much for the time being. If you can only workout at home, either buy a compact elastic band kit or get a bench with a barbell and some extra weights.

Dumbbells are a good idea, but it depends on the room you have available. I use a little of everything but for those of you on a budget, a rubber band kit really does wonders. Otherwise, with or without a barbell, squats, crunches, pushups, rear leg raises and going for a walk will work until you get that bench, barbell or rubber band kit. After the light warm-up, before you jump in and test any new exercises, I want you to next select a weight or resistance that you think allows for approximately 10 good repetitions per movement. What is a movement? An exercise. Pick one per muscle, doesn't matter what one right now.

But what exactly is a repetition? It is a single lift that consists of both a positive (or lifting) portion and a negative (or lowering) portion combined. So a rep is a one time up, and one time down motion. The amount of repetitions you perform (meaning how many times you lift a particular weight up and down again and again) per 'set' or per exercise will vary depending on your current strength, the weight you use and the goals you have. A 'set' is a collection of repetitions. If you performed 10 reps, that's a set. If you perform 2 reps, it's still a set, not a pair. A set is always going to be the complete number of repetitions you were able to perform on one exercise without stopping, doesn't matter how many that is.

I encourage you to try to do the maximum number of repetitions you possibly can each set of every exercise unless you're taking the session easy for some reason. Otherwise, I want you to work to the point of 'failure' of being able to perform another complete repetition on each set of each movement. If you do not listen to this, you will not reach your goals. And even if you can't lift the weight all the way up one more time, I want you to lower it slowly anyhow. It doesn't mean you cannot control lowering the weight even though attempts to raise it are futile.

If you have done an exercise to 'failure', and really can't perform more than you just have, the tissues have torn down to 'protect' you and prevent a continued rep. Therefore, with torn tissue, its impossible to do the same amount of reps two sets in a row. If you do 2 sets of 10, you are either not trying hard enough on the first set or you are trying much harder than you have before on the second set. Either way, it defeats the purpose. So go and attempt 15 reps next time you use a weight that allows only 10 reps on the first set. Use the same weight, try a second set, let me know if you can match those reps on the second set.

If you can, you aren't listening to me. The positive or 'concentric' lifting portion of the rep may include either pulling or pushing efforts that cause the weight selected to be lifted. Whether by cable, pulley, barbells, dumbbells or a sturdy rubber band kit, it's all the same. The raising of a weight benefits you most if you control it and take at least 4 seconds to lift. However, doing your best to control all weights so that you do not raise them faster than this is only half the battle. The other half, the negative 'eccentric' lowering motion is nothing more than the release of the weight downward towards the floor against gravity's pull.

It is considered to be the most beneficial part of the movement. This is the part of the movement that should ALWAYS be performed slowly, under as much control and released as smoothly as possible each and every repetition, especially on the very last rep you attempt to complete. 4 seconds is the fastest a rep should ever be released. That last rep should probably be released even slower. This is possible because your strength isn't in the lifting but in lowering anyhow. That's how muscle works. You'll always be able to lower more than you can lift. Lifting fights gravity, lowering works with it.

The earth is like a magnet pulling downward at your weights. Work with this magnetic effect and you will show progress in no time. We also refer to the concentric portion of the rep as either 'flexion', which is a decreasing in the angle of a joint, or the bending of a joint and 'extension' for the eccentric part which is an increasing in the angle, or the straightening of a joint. Other movements are adduction, which is the movement of a limb towards the body and abduction, which is the movement of a limb away from the body. Whatever the movement is, whatever muscle it worked, when you are done trying for more reps....

Slowly return your weight to the starting position. That is the end of your set. Now remember, I mentioned picking a weight you could lift around 10 reps with. Did you do 10? Did you not do 10? Did you do more than 10? Write it all down. Use the KNOW HOW Log Book if you aren't sure how to keep such notes. In succeeding workouts, if you notice you have become stronger on any one exercise (being able to do more than 10 reps or even more reps than that since the previous session), you must always add a little more weight to that movement the next time you train.

You do this to 'progressively' overload your ever-adapting muscles, which is what causes them to grow and your fat to burn. Letting them get used to only lifting one weight doesn't force them to work harder and that doesn't make them more efficient. So be certain to add more weight when you can handle it. If you complain of no progress, it's only because either you are not eating right or you do not try for more reps or more weight when you know darn well you should. You will keep up with this approach until your goals are met of course. After that, you can cut yourself some slack. Until then, work, work, WORK for it! So, again, if you understand what I have recommended so far, this means if you can lift a weight only 6 times, you are using too much weight.

Take some weight off or at least do not plan on adding any more weight until 10 reps are possible. If you can however lift something more than 10 times, you are not using enough weight. Add some more next time. Whether or not you are using hundreds of pounds per lift, look at this as a form of amateur bodybuilding. Listen, grandma, grandpa, you and I and any high school kid that picks up a weight is actually bodybuilding whether they like it or not. They just do not have the same goals as a professional bodybuilder.

I have no interest in being big and bulky but the same rules apply to all of us. So as soon as you can lift anything for 10 repetitions without wiggling, squirming, moving your feet, lifting one side faster than the other, making faces, holding your breath, struggling much, and doing anything else otherwise considered to be cheating to lift a weight, it's time to put a few more pounds on that machine, bar, dumbbell or even add another band to the elastic kit. For now, as soon as you've finished your set, it's time to move on to another exercise.

As you go from one movement to another in subsequent sessions, you may notice that you're only getting stronger during the first half of your workout. DON'T WORRY ABOUT THIS. It is still a sign of great progress if you maintain your strength the second half. That first half should fatigue you more than before since now you are using more weight or doing more reps. So, in your higher level of fatigue, by maintaining your strength the second half of a workout, you HAVE actually gotten stronger after all.

Anytime you maintain strength when exhausted as easily as you have in the past when rested, that's progress. Also note, some muscles are just not as strong as others and do not heal within the same time frame as the bigger ones. So be patient with your body. In the months to come, that's when you can look back and determine what worked and what didn't. I say this because you also cannot always expect to show progress from one workout to another, but from one month to the next, the results will be undeniable. But realize, to stimulate the many biochemical changes within you to make this all work, training hard is necessary but it taps deep into your energy reserves. This is the key to stimulating muscle growth and fat loss, hard work.

You do need to replenish what you depleted first thing after the session. You do not grow from the actual exercises, but from what you do to allow the healing to occur through nutrition, then rest afterwards. So please consider these factors and limit each weight training session to no more than 10 different exercises and 2 sets per muscle. That's the maximum stimulation you'll ever need. I can't remember doing more than 10 sets in one workout in a long time myself. If you want more to do, or feel one exercise per muscle isn't enough variety, you should simply change your exercises and routines every now and again.

I change my routine every 2 weeks but you could still make amazing progress only changing it every 30 days. Whatever you decide, immediately after training hard enough that you know you've stimulated your results, allow for them. Eat something. What is best to start off with? If you are a beginner, I prefer you use machines (instead of barbells or dumbbells) and fight all desire to perform more than 10 sets each session including warm ups. This goes for the experienced client too. One set to failure of ten exercises is all you need to address anyone's entire body's needs in one workout. And the entire body should definitely be worked each and every session.

After that, you eat then rest a day or so. Aerobics? You do not need as much aerobic exercise working out this way. You will experience somewhat of a cardio vascular benefit by just focusing on working harder for a change. By not reserving yourself when you train, you will experience the difference your very first session. Take notice of your heavy breathing. It's undeniably aerobic. Maybe you need more of a reason than getting to do less aerobics to perform total body workouts.

Ask any physician and they will tell you that all systems of the body interrelate and none are truly independent of another. You've read what Dr. Eversole has to say about that. The body works as a whole if healthy and it's true while being trained. The chemicals stimulated, the hormones released, the work of the blood and the lungs, they all interrelate as one system with each and every exercise you do or muscle you work. It doesn't matter how you are 'splitting' up your workouts it is still stressing to the entire human system. Do you breath differently when working legs than you do working upper back or chest muscles?

You will feel the work in the area you train but you will always breath, react and recover using the same systems of the body no matter what muscles you're singling out. If you must split the workouts into halves or thirds, at least limit the amount of exercise done to no more than 30 minutes of weights or 40 minutes total, including cardio work. More advanced body builders may require more exercises, or even an extra session at times, we are talking only one or two exercises or extra sets a muscle, not 8 or 10, just ONE or TWO.

If you train incorrectly, that's one thing, but if you train too often it will nearly always result in a loss of interest for further training, having a bad attitude about your progress. You may even have headaches that occur only while exercising, possibly diarrhea will appear between sessions, yeast infections are common in over trained women, and you'll not only be exhausted all the time but anxiety and depression over your appearance will consume you to a point you'll quit... Sound familiar? They are all effects of OVER training.

'Over training' is something that happens due to the cumulative stresses your overall supporting systems experience more so than just what happened to the particular muscles you worked on a given day. The tearing down of your biceps for example with a good set of barbell curls not only affects the nerves of the bicep, but the spinal cord they are attached to and therefore the brain. At this point the body will began trying to remedy the stress of lifting that weight and tearing of muscle by getting more oxygen coming in. That's necessary in processing more nutrients and removing waste. This is why you're breathing so heavy.

And any exercise that involves a lot of heavy breathing depletes your stamina. We can agree there. For this extremely simple and scientifically valid reasoning, it makes a heck of a lot of sense that we focus on training the entire body all in one session then letting it recover before we attempt to exercise again with minimal aerobics. "If it doesn't kill you, it makes you stronger" but the body still wasn't meant to be tortured too much or tortured everyday. The added stress of over training only increases cortisol levels, which disrupts all other positive anabolic processes that you have worked so hard to enjoy. Have I scared you from exercising at all?

The next time you have a hard time catching your breath doing something as simple as climbing stairs, maybe you'll agree you need a little more activity in your life. Are you under 18 years of age? Are you over 50? Do you experience PMS? Are you pregnant? Going bald? ALL the more reason you should begin exercising. You may need to cut the weight back a bit from what you would like to use, but you still require exercise during these important times of life more than any other.

And what we all need, even the athlete and bodybuilder, no matter how you choose to look at it, is a full body routine that tests our body's demands to stimulate results without ever over doing it. If you are a prepubescent child or anyone extremely out of shape right now who wishes to follow this exercise plan, please consult your physician and keep in touch with them until you get the hang of everything. Even though you will train on the average only 2 or 3 days a week for 20 to 30 minutes a session, it is best to have them advise you if you are currently out of shape or under 18 years of age. Getting more rest should be enough, but just in case… Talk to the doctor.

One thing is for certain, workouts this intense require more rest, so take it. This doesn't mean working out easier allows you to work out more. Easier work doesn't test you enough to do anything but maintain your appearance. We need to illicit the appropriate responses. You can potentially increase your strength by 6 times what you know it to be now following my advice but the ability to recover at most only doubles over time. What this means is you must train less often until you get stronger at first (twice a week) but once you achieve your goals, training a couple more days a week may be warranted.

Beginners can't get away with more training days for long but the experienced can train more while using heavier weights. I consider that a luxury. I can go to the gym and train, run a mile and be completely done with everything in 30 minutes 2 or 3 days a week because I am no longer looking to set personal strength records. Nothing beats that! If you are able to bench, squat, and barbell row your own weight for 10 reps minimum each, you can add an extra workout to the schedule. If not, 3 sessions a week are plenty. If you are thinking right now that aerobics must be an easier way to get started, it isn't.

Even if you are reduced to lifting feathers at first, or must cut the weight you use back to what you used as a teenager in order to perform each movement correctly, weight training is still the single most beneficial form of exercise in regards to reaching all our goals. Can you ever workout out more often than 3 times one week and 2 times the next? If you like, sure, but if you aren't progressing by getting fitter or stronger each and every session, what do you really think you'll need next? More work-outs or more rest? Remain patient with me here. If you work hard enough on at least working at increasing your weaknesses each session, but not so hard you blow a piston, even only short term, and you will get the results you seek.

Forget about entering a physique contest or becoming the Incredible Hulk right now. If that's the plan, it will happen in time. For now, focus only on your weaknesses twice a week. Do this and your weaknesses will vanish within no time and you won't worry about 3 sessions a week. I bet you're also curi-ous why I recommend only doing enough movement to break a small sweat before training. How can that be enough of a warm up to prevent injury?

When you select a weight that you think you can perform no more than 10 repetitions with under slow and controlled move-ment (remember, you're taking 4 seconds to raise the weight and 4 seconds to lower it without yanking or dropping it), by the time those ten reps are complete, a good 80 seconds should have passed. It only takes 30 seconds to properly warm a joint up. How so? If you take your time and lift a weight 4 seconds up, control lowering it down for another 4 seconds, that's 8 seconds a complete rep. After 4 reps, or 32 seconds later, enough blood has been squeezed from your working muscles into your cold and stiff tendons to 'warm' and 'loosen' them up.

This is the most natural process in protecting your ligaments and tendons. By the time the 10th rep comes around, you are probably as safe as anyone could ever hope to be as long as you aren't getting sloppy with your form. Cold tendons are like plastic, warm tendons are like rubber. If you move slow and always get the form correct before deciding to add weight to an exercise, you'll never need a formal warm up or have the pleasure of experiencing an injury. I have, and I know first hand that injuries only occur from sudden jerks like catching a refrigerator falling off a truck to save your child (Lou Ferrigno did this once).

So do not throw your weights around and you will be fine. This is why I also say it's important to get the art of movement down first or have the opinion of someone watching you, like a trainer, or a workout partner at all times. A 'spotter' is someone who guides you through the 'spots' you have trouble. You don't need to invest a lot of money in a trainer if you need one at first. The commitment is to yourself and not to the trainer. In fact, make it clear to them you are going to try one or more trainers for a session or two each so you can learn what you can about basic movements, then you plan to move on. If you doubt any one of them in any way, do not train with them any longer.

Maybe you can think of someone at work who you can ask to show you a few of the exercises mentioned in this book. Maybe you live with such a person that can help. Maybe you are related to someone who can offer guidance. If not, this is no excuse to give up. Start now by calling the gym for a one time trainer referral or look through the yellow pages. Call just one person and request just one session. Tell them you do not want a workout, you simply want them to teach you a few exercises.

From there, you will be able to build a foundation on your own. Sound simple enough? It is but it's something you requires 100% of your dedication. If you want results, I want you to clear your head of all things when you begin a movement. Concentrate on nothing else around you. The only thing that should matter while in the gym is the exercise. Block everything else out. It is essential to be in tune with your body and the motions it performs. You want to become 'one' with the task at hand and 'center' your mind along with your very existence in the experience of lifting a weight. For instance, when I work on a bicep machine, I focus on listening to my breathing from the inside and out.

I feel my biceps pulling the weight upwards while it contracts to lift and then I enjoy the feel of the handles slowly stretching the muscles as it pulls back down again lowering the weight. I pay close attention not to extend too far down or pull up too fast either. I reverse the downward movement at the exact same point each and every time to bring the weight back again too. I am aware throughout the set that my grip is not tight but relaxed. The handles or bar simply rests in the palm of my hands and is cradled as I control it. My hands are merely hooks as I feel the bicep do all my work.

I know how far up to raise the weight and I know that no one is too close to bump the bar. I see all around me without looking. I keep my head straight and I breath in and out without thought. I am not looking away from the floor for anything as I continue to focus on each repetition until I am sure one more is absolutely impossible. I never hold my breath while lifting even as the work gets harder. I keep my air passages open during all phases of the exercise to supply my body with enough oxygen to get me through the work it is doing.

Holding your breath can elevate your blood pressure to dangerously high levels and contribute to a self-induced headache. If you do begin to experience a headache while training, even a mild one, slowly return to the starting position and stop the exercise immediately. Start taking in deep breaths and develop a rhythmic pattern like you are jogging to stick with throughout each movement. Breath in and breath out several times a rep if necessary. NEVER hold it.

I try for more and more reps AGAIN AND AGAIN without flinching until I can no longer do so. The objective to training is to work harder than you did last time. That means when discomfort arises, like burning inside the muscle, ignore it. The feeling is temporary. Never stop midway. I will continue to raise the weight in 4 seconds, pause at the top barely a second just to be sure I feel the muscles are contracted, then I will lower the weight just as slowly as I raised it. If the weight seems heavier as I do more and more reps it might take 5 seconds or more to raise in those later reps. If this happens, take 5 seconds to lower it too.

It may take 6 or 7 seconds to raise and lower the weight. Once you get to the last rep, I know I must try for a full five more seconds to move the weight anyhow. Even if it only raises a hair more, I do not stop until I know for sure the weight just isn't going to budge. When I am certain the weight is not capable of being raised any further, I slowly lower the bar (which you are always capable of doing because remember, the lowering portion of a rep is where the muscle remains the strongest) and then put it back into the starting position. I stop for just a moment afterward to take a deep breath into the bottom of my lungs then get up to prepare for the next exercise. I might stretch the muscle I just worked, or I might not. But I waste no time getting to my next movement.

Slow movers have slow metabolisms. I do not rush THROUGH a set. I rush TO the set. I realize when some sets are complete, allowing for 'just' enough time to go on to the next movement may seem impossible. Not just because you must wait for someone else to get off a machine, but because working hard and trying for ten reps with something you can barely do 9 with is grueling. I have been winded for up to 15 minutes after a hard leg press or squat, but I don't stop. I move on. If you rest much longer than two minutes, you lose your anabolic edge (muscle building and fat burning potential) and your joints will 'cool' down. We don't want that to happen.

This is also why your workouts are limited to 10 sets and 10 to 12 minutes of total aerobics. No total workout should last more than 40 minutes or you're defeating the purpose of being there. You lose the hormonal boost you get from training if you 'lolly gag' around. The minute that it takes you to walk from one machine to the next is quite enough time to get mentally ready for more work. For the best results, it is important to feel completely rested and vigorous at the beginning of every workout, not necessarily between sets. Sorry, but I do not expect you to enjoy the work. I expect you to enjoy the RESULTS.

What sort of aerobics AKA…cardio work? Again, riding a bike, a rowing machine, climb a stair master, take a jog or paddle an aerodyne if you like as they all will suffice. Whichever you select, hop on your machine of choice and perform 12 nonstop minutes of serious huff and puff and don't hold back. Write down how far you travel during the exercise (150 flights of stairs, 3.5 miles, 10 kilometers, etc) and at what speed you traveled at (4 MPH of KPH, etc) in your Know How Log. If you want results, I recommend trying as hard as you can for at least 10 and no more than 15 minutes each session.

Try to achieve more distance in the same amount of time worked as often as you possibly can. I realize an average of 12 minutes doesn't seem like much but it truly is plenty for now. The reason being is that despite most people believing that after 20 minutes of cardio work your body begins fat burning, it's only true if the body has burnt it's glycogen the first 20 minutes you trained. The problem here is that the body burns a lot of amino acids (muscle) along with its glycogen during the initial 20 minutes of endurance movement. And if you keep going at it for more than 40 minutes, you'll burn even more muscle.

So while you have a 20 minute 'window of opportunity', so to speak, in the middle for fat burning after the glycogen is burned, doesn't it make sense to do something which doesn't burn muscle so all you burn is fat? That would be weight lifting! If you lift weights first you'll deplete of glycogen, preserve muscle, then when you exercise from the 20 to 40 minute time frame, you'll burn nothing but fat. However, let's assume if you're not at 10% body fat for men or 15% body fat for women yet, your body is normally 'storing' more fat than it burns.

If this is true, then your body's preferred energy sources are more than likely muscle tissues. This is why you aren't as tone as you want to be and when your fat levels are low, your muscles are fuller looking. If you grasp this concept, then you'll understand that when I say aerobics really only burn whatever your body's current preferred energy sources are for fuel, you won't want to do too much cardio work right now. If you're still fat, then those first 40 minutes of exercise (20 or 30 minutes with weights and 10 to 15 minutes of cardio) are plenty for now. Let your diet peel the fat away. Otherwise, more cardio only means you're going to stay fat. Why would you want to argue this matter? I am trying to save you time!

I do something on occasion I call HIGH intensity aerobics where I run hard as nails for 10 minutes, then I reduce my speed to 80% of that intensity for another 5 minutes. I reserve this sort of aerobics for ONLY AFTER a weight session. Occasionally upon waking, performing aerobics is good too but only if you are already able to see your abdominal muscles, but do not start such a schedule before that. And 3 days a week of

20 minutes in the morning adds up to an hour a week MAX, not an hour per session, an hour extra per week too. You will NEVER break a sweat as quickly as when doing this sort of high intensity aerobics.

Another version I made popular back in 1992 that a well known magazine ripped off from me just a few years back was where I would run for 3 minutes hard, then one minute slow, followed by 3 minutes hard, and one minute slow again for 3 complete cycles... It's AWESOME if you will do it right. Problem is, again, not many people CAN run for 3 minutes all out then only take a minute to jog at a slower pace and still be able to run another 3 minutes as fast as possible one more time. What happens is that they jog for 3 minutes then walk, then jog and that's not the point. If this is you, try the same routine on a stationary bike or rowing machine. See how it works. Finding what fits your interest is what keeps you coming back for more each session.

I use another high intensity approach to aerobic training too. The workout begins by riding my bike at a steady pace for a minute, then I increase the intensity to a higher level that has me crying to myself to quit for a full three minutes and then I go back to the easier level for a minute. Next, you guessed it, another three minutes of hard core cycling followed by one minute to cool down a little at a slower pace. Then you do this one more time and you are done.

Sounds simple but try riding at a high enough level that you'll want to quit after 15 seconds but knowing you aren't allowed to, just keep going and HATE IT but DO IT. Another cardio regime I perform involves pedaling on a bike at the lowest level for 30 seconds, which is usually Level One and increasing the levels one at a time each additional 30 second increment. Most machines go up to 12 Levels. So in six minutes, when I am at the highest level and am halfway through the 12 minute session,

I decrease one notch at a time just as I increased them. I pedal my bike as hard as my body allows until my time is up and I am back at level one again.

If you cannot make it to the top level, that is alright. Divide the time left by however many levels you completed to finish your session. If you made it to level 4 in 2 to 4 minutes, divide the remaining 8 to 10 minutes by 4, which is 2 and a half or 2 minutes and 30 seconds before you decrease the levels again. You will get it in time. Guess what. If you weight train like I suggest, you can do ANYTHING you want aerobically for these 12 minutes and you will burn fat anyhow. I look at these twelve minutes as important because they force your blood vessels to create new route openings for delivering fresh oxygen to nourish your muscle tissues.

Without this, you do not heal properly. This is what is meant by "Max VO2 uptake". It is the efficiency that oxygen is taken to the cells with nutrients to heal you. Realize, most of your life (90%) is spent performing anaerobic muscular generated movements, not aerobics. If you want to look like those fat ladies on the aerobics machines who ride, stair climb and treadmill themselves into the ground 2 hours a night and who after months still don't look any better, then sit this book down or give it away. You're not ready for the truth. Otherwise, the closer you pay attention to me, and the harder you work…

The more progress you will make. After cardio, that's when you should do some stretches, but nothing else and do not take forever about it. If I did not stretch between sets, where I normally have my partner or my 'assistant' stretch me, you can bet I did them after my workout. If I am alone, that's no excuse, I still do them by myself. I DO NOT stretch as a warm up. That's looking for trouble. Your tendons are brittle when cold. Stretch only after you've worked. It'll feel so good as the sensation of fresh blood flushes into your newly worked muscles.

In case you, your trainer or your partner do not understand stretching techniques, you may want to watch one of my video cassettes that demonstrate these procedures. After your workout, our bodies need carbohydrate foods and liquids. I suggest you have a half sized carb meal directly after the routine and a regular full sized protein meal 90 minutes following that. Not eating protein with a little fat (whey protein and cream is my choice) before a workout or having carbs afterwards then more protein 90 minutes again later will cause your body to cannibalize it's own muscle tissue. It does this looking for either recovery nutrients or the energy it needs to rebuild, otherwise defeating the purpose of the working out to begin with.

You should eat well all the time and drink plenty of water before, during AND after your workouts. But most of you are already willing to do this much. Just don't fall into the trap of having carbs before or during a workout (THAT'S REAL BAD) and waiting to eat them after. This is not good. Carbs during a session lead to dehydration, which reduces your blood volume and missing them afterwards causes you to store rather than burn fat too. So DRINK ONLY WATER and plenty of it to wash down those post workout carbs.

No matter what, you should also try to rest your body by not training at all (including aerobics) at least 48 hours between every single workout (light activity is fine on your 'off' days, but no weights are to be lifted and no tough aerobic sessions). Many people like to alternate between weights on one day and cardio-vascular exercise on the next. I would recommend against this. Rest and rest WELL. You will succeed faster. It is the resting periods between workouts that the body builds muscle and burns fat. Without sufficient rest, you make no progress.

You see, growth and fat loss do not take place until after the muscles have fully recuperated. Exercise damages you. The body requires recuperation or 'recovery' time after each session. It's healing. Like with a scab. You pick, you pick, and you bleed some more. Just let the wound heal. An EMS unit or getting a massage between sessions to speed healing is helpful but not crucial. No EMS machine is helpful in giving you amazing abs though…

Please note: When you are not at home and on the road traveling, it's all right to take an extra day off between sessions if that is what your schedule is calling for. Just make sure you get 2 sessions in a week. If you do not think you have time to get to a gym, try to make the time. Nobody, no matter how successful or busy they think they are should avoid taking a half hour to devote to a training session at least twice a week. Find a gym, get yourself to it, knock the workout off and feel good about it. Put yourself first at least twice a week. If this is impossible, then schedule a session for right before leaving town and another upon returning home. Either that or get yourself a good elastics band kit. But workout one way or another. You need it.

While we are all individuals and different, we are still all so much the same that we do not require that much more or less than the next person does, so the rules that apply to you apply to virtually anyone. In advanced cases we may take things like specific workout frequency, intensity, time, reps, environment and the type of exercise you are doing into consideration but to produce desired results, a bench press is a bench press and a row is a row and a squat is a squat. Older folk always heal more slowly. Not that 40 is old, but physical changes manifest after age 30 that tend to slow our healing a bit. If you are over 40, you better take heed. Learn to read your body. Focus. Feel each heart beat when you breath. Feel each movement you perform. Know what you are doing. Feel the stretch and contraction as you lift and lower the weights.

Come to understand any and all feedback from your body. Take notes and come to be able to instantaneously interpret feedback appropriately in order to achieve continued results. This is why you came to me. Sometimes we need to call in a driver when the road gets rough. Not that weight training is like brain surgery, but unless you create automatic habits out of these things, it's going to feel like pulling teeth just to lose or gain a pound. Like you have created bad habits over time, these are the good ones I want you to adopt today. And do not be afraid to ask for a trainer's advice if necessary.

But if their advice extends further than how to perform the exercises I recommended or differs from what you have read in this chapter so far, smile, say 'thanks anyhow' and walk away. The only thing you need to learn from anyone else now is, possibly, where a particular machine is located in the gym. The rest is within these pages. No matter your level of fitness, the only difference between most of you and the trainers you speak to anyhow is the amount of weight you use when you train.

THE ECONOMY OF EXERCISE

First thing is first, what you are about to hear is radically different from what your friends are probably doing when they work out. Keep in mind, training intensity is everything, endurance is important, recovering from a workout is foremost, speeding the metabolism and burning fat depend upon recovery… And without proper nutrition, nothing happens. The reason we can and do see results on the routines I am about to present is because we eat right. So… Are you ready to stop spinning your wheels? Then does it really matter how different what I ask you to do is? Or do you want to debate with me a while? No debate? How much more time and energy is being wasted because of IMPROPER EXERCISE TECHNIQUE and FAILURE TO MONITOR YOUR PROGRESS? Ever heard of the economy of exercise? Probably not. I think I made the term up. I came up with it because I like to do as little exercise as I have to in order to avoid doing too much in any one session and still get results. For any of us to make progress we must work hard enough to get stronger and use high intensity in our approach to get there. Think of your long-term goals at all times, not the goals of those around you.

This particular idea arose on a day that I didn't feel like waiting in line to complete my workout.

The gym was too crowded and I wasn't in the mood to deal with anyone who was hogging the machines. That day, I simply did 3 movements that covered a few muscles each and moved on. You already know you recover faster by cutting back. But to successfully pull the economy of exercise off, one would need to select only exercises that work more than one muscle group at a time to justify removing some of the other movements that don't.

We know that any work on any muscle causes stress to the entire system, but that doesn't mean all muscles are worked sufficiently by any one exercise. Because of that fact, while it's impossible to elicit maximum results training only one part of the body, you still stress your entire body with any one exercise. So why not just pick a few movements that work a bunch of muscles each and workout even less for the day?

So let's say you SQUAT. That exercise works a lot of different muscles. Some say your entire body. In reality, if you want the rest of your body worked, you must also do something like BENT OVER BARBELL ROWS if you want results in areas of the body that the squat doesn't stimulate. Most professionals would admit that this combination works a considerable amount of muscle and you really do not want to add a bunch of other exercises as they only hamper progress. Power lifters live by this rule.

While you aren't power lifting, you are looking to lift more than you do now and change the way you look, so just don't eat like a power lifter and we'll be alright. Well, since these two exercises only sufficiently hit half the upper body and all of the lower body. Squats work calves, thighs and glutes (this is the butt) while only partially working the chest, shoulders, tricep (back of the arm) and hamstrings; while rows do work the hamstrings a little, they mainly stress the upper back, rear shoulders, forearms and biceps) so you must also do BENCH PRESSES to make up the weak links (chest, front shoulders and triceps). That is how you pick out three exercises.

From here, you might perform 2 warm ups for squats and one each for rows and benches, but that's only 7 total sets in your workout. I often stop right here. What if the entire system is stressed so much during that it couldn't possibly recover fast enough for you to workout again on schedule? Is it a revolutionary approach I suggest you also take? Can it be possible that all our goals can be reached using just 3 exercises? 7 sets? Why not? It is at least possible. It worked for me and it WILL work for you. Think what you like, but I built one client's upper back, chest and legs to a point that many would have thought years of training were required. However, in less than six weeks, on a program of 5 workouts every 2 weeks of 20 minutes each, magic occurred.

He gained over twenty pounds of overall body weight, increased his arms two inches each, reduced his waist by 2 inches and increased his strength enormously. His wife, also a client on the 3 exercise system, dropped 4 dress sizes, took 1 1/2 inches off her arms, 4 off her hips and worked out even less than her hubby. She didn't need the warm-ups so she performed just THREE SETS a workout. I am NOT exaggerating. No drugs, no fat burners, no two hour-long workouts, and nothing secret. Just a simple routine of three very basic exercises and following the Know How diet plan. Another 3 exercise combo that works wonders are Leg Presses, Standing Military Presses, and Underhand Grip Pull downs.

No extra movements of any kind were added that time either, and even with my most advanced pupils, absolutely nothing else was done except for 3 sets of 3 exercises for a total of 9 sets plus 12 minutes of cardio afterwards 2 or 3 times a week. We tried Leg Presses, Underhand Grip Pull Downs or Rows and Bench Presses. Total symmetry was achieved in all clients doing any combination. Not realistic? I was personally on these routines for a full year. When you meet me, I am not as big as a body-builder like I was when that was my plan, but you can judge for yourself if I look like all I do is chest, back and leg exercises.

All I can say is that our results far surpassed the results ever obtained on any other program over any other time frame. If that weren't true, I wouldn't be including it in this book. Besides, if the other celebrities, pro fitness, modeling, elderly, teenage, male and female clients I have had on abbreviated workout routines can succeed, why can't you? What makes you so different? Are you from Mars? You can never be much like any one else. Despite any of us needing a little shaping up, I am sure you are just fine as you are. We all have plenty of potential for physical excellence despite poor physical condition. Allowing ourselves to get out of shape is the same thing as getting ourselves into shape. It's decision making, not genetics. Try what I suggest and you will experience THREE TIMES THE RESULTS IN A FOURTH THE TIME! So get on it! On the average, a 30 pound fat loss for women required just 4 hours and 38 minutes TOTAL exercise over 7 weeks! Men on the other hand were gaining 25 pounds in 7 weeks with just 5 hours and 12 minutes of TOTAL EXERCISE! Ladies, this means women require less exercise to achieve a similar result!

Remember, I earlier stated that all you needed was one exercise per muscle group for up to 10 sets a workout and maybe a few more sets or an extra workout if you are an advanced case. So none of that has changed. If you did 3 sets of 3 exercises then that would be 9 sets. Do something for your stomach and you've got ten. Do 3 sets on one exercise and 2 for 2 others and you have 7 sets total. Add one set of 3 other exercises if you feel you should. Or, do as I recommend, start with the minimal amount of work and see how much you really need to show results.

You've ready my book, you've seen my work, you've heard my interviews. I am not crazy. So what if this works? Do not be discouraged to try this by my making statements about my becoming so strong on some movements I needed to switch to others. My point is that you may never get that strong so you could in fact use these movements quite a long time if you like. One client spent two months only dead lifting and benching. Nothing else. His dead lifting went from 225 pounds for 10 reps to easily handling 405 pounds for 12 reps. His bench went from 225 for 4 to 315 for 8 reps in the same time span. A friend's 16 year old daughter got plenty stronger as she dropped well over 40 pounds in 63 days eating 2000 calories a day performing only incline chest presses and walking dumbbell lunges 3 days a week.

Ladies, I know you don't really like being in the gym around all those men. But since you will only need to do 3 exercises twice a week and spend barely 5 to 15 minutes doing them from now on, just do it. The weight loss you will stimulate is amazing. The secret to fat loss is not in how many calories you burn while exercising or how many calories you neglect to eat in order to force yourself into a deficit. The secret is in how many calories you burn the other 23 hours and 30 minutes that day and in the next 24 hours or so that you spend without exercising on your off days.

Fat burning is regulated by how much muscle you carry. Muscle burns calories for your body to use as energy and fat does nothing but look bad. The more muscle, even if it is just a little more, that you have, the more fat you will naturally burn while doing nothing. The purpose of a workout is to fatigue your muscles, not to just lift the weight to go through the motions. No matter the person, no matter the goal, you must try to work as hard as possible (within the limitations of safety) every time you train to force the body to become better, tougher, stronger, leaner and more attractive. If you want to look like those fat ladies on the aerobics machines 2 hours a night who after months still don't look better, then sit this book down or give it away.

Otherwise, the harder you work, the more progress you make. Only three core exercises. One set of each is all you need. In fact, if rest between exercises is limited ideally, you can complete a total body workout in as little as TEN minutes. Adequate rest between workouts is essential, adequate rest between exercises is only required to take as long as it takes to get from one exercise to the next as conveniently as possible. The seconds it takes you to walk to the next machine or unload your barbell is enough time to get ready for the next set.

Your friends will doubt this is true at first. But who will have more free time on their hands? You or them? Do not look back for the next three months and THEN you should go back and see what they have to say. You'll be LIGHT YEARS ahead of them. If they know so much, wouldn't they be further ahead than they are as it is anyhow?

The next chapters cover how to perform the core exercises, which I feel belong in almost any routine, but most importantly, in an economical workout plan. The only argument I have received against this sort of routine is that you are not providing your body with a balance.

Then after the same nay sayers tried it for a month, they reported back. They can't believe how effective it actually was. And you really will gain more strength than you ever thought possible too. Test your barbell curls after a month and you'll see. In fact, most all the other movements you test will show strength increases.

I have found one drawback with a program like this and that is that the weights you use might become so heavy that your joints actually become sore. It doesn't require 600 pounds on your back to be stressful to the joints. If this occurs, you are either strong enough, need more rest between sessions or you are not working out properly. Since I am not looking you in the eye to tell you this, you decide which applies to you… People do not believe me that I drive BY not TO the gym, drop by, do one set of 3 exercises then go about my business elsewhere but hey, do I really care what they believe? I am the one who looks his best with little effort….

BENT OVER ROWS AND PULL DOWNS

Bent Over Rows can produce plenty of fat burning muscle, greater upper back development leading to a more tapered waistline, and works you hard enough in just one set that you can't help but burn some fat afterwards. This covers it all and discusses why we all need to do them. Rows, seated on a machine, cable or using a dumb bell, are considered 'compound' exercises because they incorporate more than one muscle group when you perform them.

The muscles worked are the ones which run on the outside of the mid back (from, around and near the spine), your hamstrings (back of your thighs), your upper mid back (the rhomboids), the lats (on the back of the ribs), the front of your upper arms (biceps), your forearms and even the anterior (back) part of your shoulders. This exercise works a good 1/3 of the body if not more all by itself. If your lower body and back are already in good shape, you can easily handle impressive weights while performing rowing exercises.

I would suggest doing them with dumbbells, one side at a time, if you're a beginner. Don't brush off the use of dumbbells for this exercise. Working one arm at a time certainly won't SHRINK your muscles. However, as with any rowing motion, you need to carefully monitor your lower back while sticking with the best possible 'form' you can. 'Form' means 'technique' by the way. What I mean here is that your lower back should be kept flat, your shoulders held back, head high and never let your mid back rotate downward at any point in the movement. The weight should be held at arms length, always remaining several inches from the floor. An under hand grip is used on the barbell with your palms up. With dumbbells, the palm faces the body.

If you use a barbell the weight is pulled into your belly button, not your chest. If you use a dumbbell, row it to your hip bone and bring that elbow high behind the ribs. The other elbow will be propped up on the knee of the same side while the working arm handles the weight straddled between your legs. Your knees are always kept slightly bent, sturdy and solidly in place.

No dipping, swaying or standing. Let one arm or both arms do the work. No matter what, do not row to the chest. Row high enough that you feel your shoulder blades squeezed back together and contracted for a moment before lowering the weight again to a straight arm position.

This movement should precede the bending of your arms. Then, when the arms do pull the weight in to your body, you really crimp your muscles together for a full contraction. Next in importance is making sure the weight doesn't touch the floor or if you use a machine, the plates on the cable do not come together until the set is done. You need a full range of motion as they say, all the way in, all the way out when lifting. While seated, rowing machines provide full-ranges of motion, machines with padding at your chest remove the stress involved on the lower back and legs. You need this stress to some extent to stimulate results.

For this reason, machines are not as effective in stimulating overall growth as barbell or straddling dumbbell rows. I used a plate loading machine one year while bodybuilding when I became TOO STRONG at rows for my lower back to keep up with the main muscles. I was rowing 450 pounds on a barbell and using 250 pounds with a dumbbell. I hadn't any other choice. If you aren't that strong, then stick with a barbell or dumbbell. No matter the strength, do only two sets maximum when rowing. One to warm up and one to failure as explained earlier. If you need a second warm-up, have one, but do not exhaust yourself with the effort.

Do not exceed three sets total and only make one of them your hard working set. Each session, be sure you add more reps or weight as prescribed and if you have a weak lower back due to disease or injury, a padded rowing machine is fine. I mostly perform pull downs these days. They work the same upper back muscles, force the biceps to support the movement more but do not affect the lower body at all. I like them because they also stretch my spine upward which is extremely important for nervous system health. Rows and pull downs have an endless number of variations, but each must follow the same rules as the others to ensure that the upper back gets proper stimulation. However, with pull downs, you don't squeeze the shoulder blades together in the middle.

You rotate the chest up towards the bar and the blades downward. These movements start from a hanging position where you will feel a full stretch down the sides of your upper back. I use an underhand grip here as well. That's a 'palms facing you' grip. From the hanging position, with my hips completely under the 'knee' pads, sitting as close to them as possible or directly under the pulley overhead, I pull by shrugging my shoulders down (where they stay throughout the movement) and rotate them back. I focus on pulling my entire body to the bar even though the bar is really coming to my body.

I pause with my elbows situated behind me, so to speak, before raising the weight just to the point my arms are straight again. I do not reach upward so my shoulders feel the stretch and the weight plates do not touch together until the set is done. If you do not row or do pull downs all the way in to the body and spread the shoulder blades back at the end of the movement, the mid back goes unaffected. If you stretch too far upward at the top, you are doing further shoulder work to pull it back down in order to work your back at all again.

Add it all together with extra military presses and flyes and no wonder your shoulders look so much more developed than your back and chest does. You aren't working your chest and back! Only shoulders! 3 sets maximum, 2 are warm-ups.

1 set is still to this day all I perform. If I need a warm-up set, I tend to go to other exercises. Once you're strong enough, you

need that extra set. You do not need to become much stronger in my opinion.

I can go 6 months without exercising and still be able to sit down on a pull down machine and use the entire weight stack. If you are at this level, you might want to look into one of those leather belts, which has a chain hanging from it. The chain is used to loop additional weight to your body so that the exercise isn't so easy.

TIP: Wrist straps are NOT to be used. Unless you are a power lifter, do NOT use them. If you are using wrist straps because of a weak grip, then get rid of the wrist wraps and let your hands strengthen up. Worst thing that could happen is that you become so strong your wrists cannot row or dead lift something.

If that's the case, you're strong enough and need alternative exercises. In a matter of weeks, you will see and feel the difference as well. I have trained over half my life and to this day can lift weight most people haven't an interest in achieving but I have never needed wrist straps to achieve such feats.

If you suffer lower back pain from doing rows or any other exercise, first consider whether you are exercising correctly. Slow movement, body position, etc. If so, contact a physician for a checkup.

MILITARY PRESSES AND BENCH PRESSES

We're talking about the simple bench press or standing overhead press. They are two of the best exercises for gaining pure overall upper body development and strength. Dumbbell side lateral raises can be used to address different parts of the shoulders and dumbbell flyes or 'pec' deck machines work other parts of the chest if desired, but it is the standing press we really ought to start off with. The standing overhead 'military' press works on the muscles of the upper chest, neck, shoulders, and back of the upper arms (triceps) too.

We usually do them standing to also work the legs and calves but this isn't why we suggest barbells. Most shoulder machines force you to perform the exercise in an odd manner that over stretches the shoulder joint and increases the risk of rotary cuff injuries. You don't want that. Simply stand in a squat rack with a barbell right in front of you. Have the bar at chest height, place your palms on it facing forward, keep your elbows in towards your ribs, not flared away, and pick up the bar. Start with it resting on your collar bone then step away from the rack.

Keep your feet shoulder width apart and planted firmly on the ground with both knees bent just a little. Do not squat, dip or kick. Stand completely still. Look to the ceiling and press the bar upward until your arms are straight above your head without reaching any higher. Without pausing, lower the barbell back to the starting position at your collar bone again. Repeat until you cannot perform another rep. Stop, then rest. Do only 2 sets. One is a warm up, or if you're strong, maybe you'll need 2. But that's a maximum total of 3 sets. Anymore and you will over train. I used a special machine for pressing one year but I got so strong, I began to actually bend at the spine under the weight and it really got uncomfortable.

I had to go back to the barbell but once I got to a point of lifting my bodyweight over my head for 10 repetitions, I realized it was time to do INCLINE BENCH PRESSES instead. This switch took a tremendous amount of pressure off my spine. But once my strength increased to using one and a half times my body weight for 10 reps, I moved over to performing regular BENCH PRESSES. After a while there, I felt stagnant so I moved over to the seated plate loading chest machine. You too can make these transitions as you progress based upon your better interests. If the military press isn't developing your chest, shoulders and triceps, move to the incline, then the bench, then the machine.

Now keep two more things in mind, when I say machine, you need something that handles more weight than you can use on barbells. And I also suggest you use a chest press machine if you are over 40 anyhow. It's better on your blood pressure. The second point is that there is no need for you to move from one exercise to the other any sooner than a month between each. Like I said, I have done a handful of movements for a full year while making more progress than I had using a variety of exercises. So don't get over zealous. Pick something and stick with it for a while. MAKE SURE you get results by putting your ALL into it.

You will no doubt need some work on all of these exercises to develop a nice chest, but despite thinking you need to be genetically gifted to become really fit looking, that's just not true. It's work. If you want it, work for it, and it will happen. Many people call the flat bench press the squat of the upper body. The most important thing to remember about the bench press, incline press or using a chest press machine is that you start with your arms straight but you do not raise the shoulders off the bench.

The shoulder blades must be rotated back and squeezed together behind you at all times. This pushes the ribs and chest up higher or forward. More muscle is stretched and used when the bar or machine handles comes down as your arms bend from such a position. The simple task of not reaching upward but merely straightening the arms to raise your weight is the most effective tip for developing your chest. If you raise your shoulders off the bench when you press, you aren't working your chest. That's shoulder work. Especially if you do not lower the bar all the way down either.

Imagine raising the bar up to the top, locking your arms then raising the bar higher towards the ceiling. That extra raise you do is all shoulder work. And by not lowering the bar to your chest, you aren't sufficiently stretching the pectoral muscles to recruit chest fiber for growth. As to whether you lower the handles or bar to your neck or use a wider grip isn't as important as being sure to keep the elbows away from your ribs at all times. Take a slightly wider than shoulder width grip if you are taller and a narrower grip if you're a shorter person but never grasp the bar narrower than your shoulder width. Use this same grip rule on incline and standing presses.

On a bench or on a machine, place your feet firmly on the ground and do not move them. This will stabilize you for the rest of the movement. You must arch your back as previously stated to keep the shoulders back, but you are required to keep your buttocks on the bench or seat at all times. When lowering the weight, never bounce it off your chest. Use a touch and go technique where the bar or handles are taken down slowly, making contact with the chest and just as lightly, until it is fully extended.

Throughout the movement, do not grip the bar hard. Let it rest in the palm of your hand like a sturdy ledge. Too tight of a grip will restrict the other muscles being used. Remember, we want each muscle group to have a good workout. If you push or pull a compound exercise to a point the larger muscle gives up and you feel your arms shaking trying to pick up the slack, you're on your way in the right direction my friend. But if your smaller muscles give out first, odds are you're gripping the weight too tight. Hands are for resting, leveraging, hooking a weight, not clenching and leaving impressions on the bars.

Make your impression on the rest of the body. Not your gripping power. That comes naturally in time. When you bench press, you should always keep the shoulders back into the bench and only reach as high as extending the elbows. Straighten the arms, but do not reach for the ceiling. The shoulders DO NOT leave the bench. For the greatest overall chest development, I would perform only incline bench presses. Raise the foot platform, the seat or lower part of the machine higher if you 'have to' in order to get the correct angle. While lying back, you should be somewhere halfway between upright and flat if you are on an ideal incline.

Keep your elbows flared out away from your body too, NOT in towards your ribs as you move the weight, but away from you. Lower the bar to touch just below your collar bone, NOT lower, NOT higher. A third exercise you could rotate in and out of your schedule is the Parallel Bar Dip. You can do these possibly using a dip belt (leather belt with a chain to strap weight to your body) or a machine if dips without added weight are tough for you. Many people can only do dip movements on a machine, which is fine. Whether on a rack or on a machine, do not let your elbows get higher than your shoulders or you will encourage shoulder pain. The regular dip, performed between two parallel bars in an upright position, is a superb exercise.

Going too deep only leads to potential joint pain and damage in the shoulders, elbows and wrists. Weaker people may want to only practice "negative-only dips" until they are strong enough to do them properly. I advise this, actually. Starting from the top position, slowly lower down, then climb back to the top again without trying to lift yourself. If you have already suffered from shoulder injuries, dips are not recommended until you've fully rehabilitated. I will not go into how to perform them because I do not want to encourage the beginner to do something they haven't received hands on guidance in. I'd rather you get a trainer to show you.

Are you beginning to get the idea that your training goals should be aimed more towards things we have discussed today as opposed to what you've been doing? Combine the 1, 2, or 3 sets performed for chest, shoulders and triceps with your 1, 2, or 3 sets of Rows or Pull downs and you will have done only 2, 4, or 6 total sets so far. Sometimes, I perform just a 2 set superset for chest on the Hammer Strength Iso Lateral Chest Press Machine.

Depending on my mood and how energetic I'm feeling that day, I will sit down with a good 180 pounds on the rack. Without stopping for a break, moving the weight 4 seconds up and 4 seconds down, I do my best to complete 30 reps. Some days I can, some I can't but I do try as hard as possible to make sure I reach the point of not being able to do another rep. Without rest, my partner slaps on another 100 pounds and I do another set. No rest. How? It's a different set of muscle fibers being used. Same muscle, different fibers. You may be able to use more or less weight but try this sometime. Surprise yourself.

LEG PRESSES AND SQUATS

I first used squats as my sole lower body exercise, but I noticed as I got stronger, it was too much stress on my lower back to Row AND Squat on the same day. Does squatting hurt your back? Adjust your technique or move on to the leg press. If you aren't using your own bodyweight across your shoulders to squat yet, it's your technique, not the weight. In my prime, I could use 405 pounds for 20 reps squatting. Couple that with the same weight on rows and it was just too much for my back. That's when I switched to Leg Presses. I loved the results I got too. And every time I turned anyone else over to LEG PRESS-ES, their overall muscle mass and fat loss shot through the roof BIG TIME as well.

Try this the next time you workout. Get on the leg press after adjusting the chair's height to a comfortable position. Sit so your body is at a 90 degree angle. Not too far back, nor forward. Put your feet high enough that when your legs are straight, they form a 90 degree angle with your hips and shoulders. If not, sit the seat back a little more. Once adjusted, point your toes out JUST A WEE bit. Get up and add enough weight you can only do about 10 reps. Once loaded, sit back down.

Breath deeply several times a rep and do ten straight reps. Count them in your head. 1, 2, 3, 4, 5, 6, 7, 8, 9, and 10 in the usual slow pace and do not stop until you reach 10. Pause for a moment but do not re-rack the weight. Keep it up. Look up at a mark on the high wall in front of you or at the platform itself while pushing these reps out but do not EVER look down. Also do not round or hunch your back forward as you want your breathing passages open, not restricted. Lower the weight only about half of the way down.

Do not bounce out of the top or bottom position. You're only lowering 6 to 8 inches or so and never straightening your legs so much they bend backwards on these movements. And I know I said stick with 10 reps on all exercises, but with legs, 20 good reps are marvelous for shaping the muscle. Why? Legs are designed for a little more endurance. So perform 4 more reps no matter how much it burns you then pause at the top again without bending your knees backwards and take a deep breath before doing 3 more reps and pausing again. This doesn't mean you hold your breath for these extra reps. You're simply taking an extra one before moving on. 10 plus 4 plus 3 more is 17 reps so far.

You need to do 3 more and you're done. When you complete rep number 17, do not give in and tell yourself that you'll do 20 next time. DO it now. The squat will test your will. Only quit if you cannot complete that rep. Next time, finish it, don't sell yourself short. Going easy is what's gotten you here. Don't wait to find the best foot position for you while the weight is up off the rack. Holding the weight up on one leg to find the position for the other is a fast way to get hurt. Also, do not place your feet at any extremes (like facing them too far inward as a penguin would or too far out like a duck). You are neither a penguin nor a duck.

Make sure you keep yourself flexible by stretching your hamstrings after this exercise (actually after all three of these exercises). This is important because you're technically performing this movement in a bent over position. This causes the periformis muscle to crimp around your sciatic nerves. If you do not stretch the hamstrings and possibly the glutes afterwards, it leads to weak knees eventually. Squatting and leg presses do not cause knee problems like patella tendonitis.

Walking on an incline, jumping up and down, running awkwardly and using bad form are what cause bad knees! Bet you didn't realize that! This is why we only lower the weight part of the way down too. The fact you are bent over and the way the muscles behind the knee connect, you have a natural stretching effect that's causing another natural contraction of all the muscles from your heels to your hips. That is what makes this such a marvelous exercise, but dangerous if you lower the weight too far. Over time, you will feel the difference.

And do not wear knee wraps because if you actually do need them to perform, then it's probably too much weight to begin with. I know you are cheating if you are using them. If you can't handle the weight without them, lower the weight you use. Again, we have these exercises and stretches on video if you are interested. Squats are still a great exercise to perform, but I really feel unless you are competing in athletics, leg presses are more than sufficient. I squat every now and again because it's such a natural movement, like sitting in a chair, but I do not use nearly as much weight as I once did.

I squat now solely for flexibility. In fact, the year I was bodybuilding and weighed well over 260 pounds, all I did was leg press. Well, I added leg curls every now and again, but doing only 2 sets of leg presses a workout followed by a set of high rep leg curls suited me fine. I didn't add several sets as I didn't want to over train. Women tend to avoid both leg presses and squats because they fear bigger hips and thighs but in reality, only poor eating habits will cause that to happen. I honestly feel everyone needs to learn how to squat. At least practice them once in a while. Squatting requires you to control your balance, acuity, flexibility, and patience. It's the same as standing from a chair without assistance.

For some, this is tough enough. For others, you'll require a barn on your shoulders to produce results. No matter the weight you use if any at first, realize there is a direct correlation between discomfort experienced while performing things we aren't used to and attaining the best results. If you are new to this, practice squatting without a barbell. Stand upright, feet flat, facing the same direction you would if you were walking with feet shoulder width apart. Raise your hands straight out in front of you and hold your finger tips as high as your eyes. Keep your heels on the ground. If you lean forward, your knees go over your toes, and your heels will come up.

Leaning forward shifts muscle emphasis from the legs to the back. Suck your midsection in (abdominal muscles) because that's what's keeping you erect anyhow. Often, the midsection is as weak as the rest of you due to neglect but it's possible to regain its strength by simply sucking it in every time you exercise. Keeping the butt back and down with your shoulders and head up will also remedy this for you. So as you squat down, think of it as sitting back into a chair, only the chair isn't there. Stare at a spot on the wall in front of you about a foot higher up than you are tall. As you squat down, keep your eyes, head and finger tips up.

Go down low enough that you could sit a coffee mug on your thigh and it wouldn't fall. Your thighs will be parallel to the floor in this position. Do not give in to the temptation of raising your heels. If you point out your toes in the wrong direction you will misalign the femur, tibia/fibula and foot joints. This grinds away at your tendons between the bones and pulls ligaments from their foundations. Soreness isn't always a good thing folks. Hard work is essential. Injury is avoidable. At first, you may not even be able to squat all the way down and come back up one time.

With practice, that one time will become 20 if you stick with it. And whether you use weight or not, the development will be undeniable. Expect to see a significant increase in leg definition within just a few sessions. But to keep results coming, once you're finally being able to perform 20 repetitions straight, it's time to place a bar across your shoulders but below the neck bones. Add weight each session to your bar if you're achieving 20 reps and always use spotters. You want to be sure you aren't sacrificing technique in the process of adding weight. You do not force results that way. Results come when you train properly.

Check yourself in the mirror as you squat if no one is there to guide you and please do your squats inside of a squat rack or between two sturdy items that allow you to raise and lower yourself with a place to stop if you can't regain the standing position. Lower yourself from wherever you are stuck and set the weight down. Walk away. Listen to your body. All you really need besides this advice is listening to your body. The slightest shift in your center of gravity during a squat can ruin the entire set. As you may of noticed, I haven't gone too in depth about injury and rehab.

If you happen to have areas of concern or joints of your body that hurt from a previous injury, simply go light with the weights until they feel better. I have suffered 3 injuries outside of the gym that caused me to suffer while training or pursuing results in the gym and rushing the healing doesn't benefit anyone. Each incidence took me several months of light exercise in order to rehabilitate. It was frustrating becoming somewhat inactive, but since you should always be eating right, you won't get fat during down time, and in fact, you might make progress in other areas if you're clever about it.

You can still allow for healing to occur and get to workout by just cutting the weight you use back, sometimes dramatically. That's what a therapist will have you do anyways you know. I always came back stronger as soon as I healed. It was almost like I 'needed' a break. So please consult a medical professional if something out of the ordinary occurs to you before heading to the gym in pain. Should you wear a weight lifting belt? I don't know. I feel if you wear a belt you tend to get too relaxed and most people end up pushing their bellies out into the belt thinking it still somehow protects them from injury. That's the fastest route to a hernia.

It is only when you train without a belt, using your mind as a guide, that you discover whether you really need a belt or not. You sure wouldn't push your guts out with no belt on would you? No. You'll suck it in, move more carefully, lift slowly, watch what you are doing, and be certain not to do anything too crazy, won't you? I say unless you are power lifting or working in a ballistic manner (Why would you ever do that to begin with?), there is no need for a belt. Again, working without one is why we really don't need to do much in the way of abdominal exercise.

The sucking in, holding still, maintaining good posture, and making of simple movements from start to finish in any given exercise is going to strengthen you up more than any abs class anywhere from Los Angeles to New York! And I mean that! We will cover why this is true and what to do if you really do have weak abdominals in my Personal Trainers Business Guide. What I want you to understand with this chapter is that you really only need to do 3 foundation exercises to succeed in your training. More isn't always necessary. Beginners may want to use machines that help them get familiar with general movement, but after that....

If you do one set of each either leg presses or squats, pull downs or rows, bench or military presses, and you do your sets correctly, you can add a few sets for arms, calves, or whatever else. Just do not add more than the recommended total sets per session, and I really wouldn't see it as a problem. If this confuses you, don't let it. Do one exercise per muscle group and follow the rules of gauging when it is time to add weight or if you are using too little or too much to start. I break the body down when I train into areas of: Shoulders, Hamstrings, Thighs, Biceps, Triceps, Chest, Upper Back, and maybe a set of Abdominals. But just one set of each is plenty. I cannot repeat myself often enough on this matter.

And follow your diet. Exercise does not replace a bad diet because exercise burns bodily fuels more than it will ever burn food fuels. Food has to be processed and stored before it's used as energy. I use the Know How diet and the same approach discussed in this chapter in my training today and my training back in the 'day' so to speak. After a while of following these rules, I was muscular and weighing over 270. While it wasn't just diet that got me so big, it was training, I exercised HARD EVERY SESSION to bring on all that muscle. You may only need to work hard and gain 5, 10, 15 or 20 pounds of muscle. Once you do, you will only work to maintain your results.

I at one point had other goals. And if I could reach my goals, which were fantastic, then building 5 to 20 pounds of additional muscle to replace 5 to 20 pounds of additional fat that you do not need, really isn't so tough to accomplish. You make the call. You control the results. But the path to success is the same for any of us. And part of that success will come faster if you stretch your muscles AFTER not before you workout. We demonstrate the stretches in our videos as not to lend confusion to something laid out in print. More on that in a bit…

What is a really intense workout like if all you have are a few exercises to do? Try doing a set to failure one any muscle with a weight that allows barely 12 repetitions without cheating. The second you fail on that final rep, add 25% more weight and go again without rest. You will only be able to perform possibly 4 to maybe 8 repetitions but I want you to slowly squeeze them out anyhow. Afterwards, once failure is reached a second time, drop to half the weight you started with and go again. I have seen people perform anywhere from only 10 repetitions to as many as 30 repetitions with this 'lite' set so test yourself, see what you can do. When completed, stretch that muscle slowly into a deep position and hold it, breathing in and out like a runner, stretching a little further on each breath, for a total of 60 seconds. Tell me once you have done this that you have ever performed something so intense and I will shake your hand. You won't be able to!

This will be the most brutal session of exercise you have ever done but because you are taking your supplements, eating a lot of food and getting rest while taking days off between sessions, you have nothing to fear. The better your nutrition, the better you can and will not only train but perform and see results.

Also note, a training partner is important but I would rather train alone on machines than with someone who doesn't have the same interest, drive, attention span or communication skills as I do. They will waste my time at best.

Many people consider themselves hardgainers, actually, most people do, but in reality, you're just not eating enough or correctly, plain and simple. You can try all the killer workouts you like to put on the mass but if you are still a hard gainer, you and I both know one thing is true, you should feed yourself better.

Forced reps, never do them, not necessary. Getting assistance to complete your last rep on a set is one thing, doing them over and over, a waste of precious energy. Negatives, wouldn't bother. You're asking for trouble and waiting much too long between sessions to recover. Supersets, where you go from one set without rest to another, I advocate their use daily. I do not believe in resting beyond what you truly must in order to perform each and every following set from my second to my last. Your body is there to work, not take a vacation. The only rest I take is to stretch a muscle before moving on to the next one. If I am doing two exercises for the same muscle, I do not rest. If it is two sets of the same exercise, 30 to 90 seconds is plenty enough time to take a break. Anything more, you are being lazy…

If you do as I ask, you will become more flexible, have better endurance, become much stronger and will everyone you know is going to compliment you not only on how you look but your new found confidence.

The reason people you admire succeed is not because they are good, special, chosen or even proper role models. No, it is because they have the mental acuity, the mind set, the drive, passion and commitment to push themselves past their own limitations each and every chance they get.

I would be lying if I didn't say that most people I see in the gym sacrifice form to use weight they cannot handle safely and they are not making the progress they would like to either. For instance, when you bench press, be aware of the muscles in your back working at the same time. When you curl a barbell, be aware of your triceps working at the same time. If you focus on your opposing muscles, you will notice the ones being directly trained pushing or pulling ever stricter.

It is imperative you use slow and strict motions when both lowering and raising a weight on all reps. Think the rep through, be certain of the action. Bring the weight to your body and just when you are about to lock out a rep before going again, slowly turn the movement around without straightening your limbs or losing control.

I believe every body needs to perform high rep exercises as well as aerobics to build up their cardiovascularity most efficiently. Aerobics force oxygen, which carries nutrients, throughout the body and a high level of cardio health increases both the number and size of your blood vessels. You benefit in the form of speeding the metabolism through nourishment, improved oxygen uptake which burns fat and you will even clean the body of waste easier. The key is not to do your sessions starving as many recommend before breakfast but to do them brief and hard like everything else we have discussed. Exercise can not be considered effective if you aren't gasping for air at least a little bit. Push your thresholds, do not allow yourself to remain the same and you won't remain the same.

KNOW HOW AEROBICS

One day a man somewhere between the age of 40 or 45 walking into a martial arts academy and expressed an interest in taking some lessons. He began watching the class for a little while and notices that some of the 'senior' students look very relaxed and appear to be enjoying themselves immensely, while some of the ' newer' students are straining, red faced, stressed, tense and quickly exhausted. He calls the instructor over to the viewing area and asks why there is such a dramatic difference between the two groups. He goes on to state that he has come in today because he had seen one of the guys from class over at the local gym and pointed out that this kid was in pretty good shape. "But shouldn't he be able to outlast these other guys?" he asks.

Now before I tell you what was explained to him, I would like to clarify a few things first. The Know How is not a program that is against methods of aerobic training like stationary bicycles, tread-mills, stair climbers, etc. These machines and even their counter parts i.e. mountain bikes, running stadium stairs or going for a jog all have their place and there are even scientific formulas that one can use to meet goals we never could without them. I simply choose to tell this story to those of you who possibly don't see yourselves using the above-mentioned apparatus to achieve those goals.

I think many of us would like to know how else to incorporate some aerobics into our training and benefit from other activi-ties/hobbies that we enjoy, rather than simply doing aerobics for the sake of doing them. Let's get back to the story shall we? The man who saw this other young fellow excelling on the aero-bic machines at the fitness club also saw that same young guy this night run completely out of gas and become completely exhausted in a matter of minutes wrestling!

It's all about 'functional' strength he was told. He looks at the instructor a little confused and says "Isn't that what the lifting of weights is for?" Yes and no. The conversation goes on to give him an everyday example of the differences like when you go to carry your groceries out of the store. Assuming you're not too lazy and just push one of those carts, then you will notice that from your "weight training" they don't seem as heavy as they used to. You're stronger. He agrees. However, did you also notice that after you've carried them all the way to the end of the parking lot that they did still seem ALOT heavier the further you carried them and you are now winded too? He smirks like he relates to what he is hearing. This is the difference between functional strength and aerobic conditioning!

A senior student comes over to ask something, and it became clear to both of them that the student had been working hard and that his heart rate was elevated. His deep, heavy breathing gave that away. No calculations of 220 minus your goat's age and dividing by how many eggs you eat were even necessary to arrive at the conclusion he was working hard. This student had been using EVERY muscle in his body for a wrestling session that lasted about 15 minutes or so. The coach told the visitor that by training in this particular martial art, you end up doing any sort of a combination of bends, twists, kicks, pulls, shoves, holds, pins, etc that are performed repetitiously enough to become the equivalent of doing aerobics. Not Tae Bo…

Coupling this sort of aerobic training WITH demanding exercises at a gym brings about a functional strength level that indeed exceeds that of spending hours on a stair stepper because it carries over to many of our daily activities. Yes, like carrying groceries to the car. How often in life will you be required to run for 3 hours? Not often.

But those bursts of energy to do house work, carry groceries, they pop up often, but they aren't half as tough as going all out for 15 minutes at a time, are they? The instructor could see that he was looking at the class in a completely different way now.

He was beginning to understand that aerobics didn't have to be done on a bike, or a rowing machine and that doing them on a machine may not help him do the things that HE does regularly any better. There is no flexibility involved, no variation in movement... Suddenly martial arts became realistic, in a functional sort of way.

Aerobics should play an important role in your life. To feel more alive, have more energy and add quality time to your schedule are reasons enough to at least cut back. Interestingly enough, there have been substantiated studies that prove deep diaphramatic or 'deep' breathing practiced regularly can actually have as much if not more effect on the cardiovascular system than running on a treadmill for 30 minutes!

Sounds strange doesn't it? If we think about why we do cardio to begin with, it is to increase the amount of oxygen that is taken into our bloodstream. Deep breathing is what rapidly increases this factor. We do aerobics just to stimulate fat loss through deeper breathing. That's all. We are forced to do this because most of us are shallow (or chest) breathers almost all the time. We need to breath into our bellies, our diaphragms, if we want our lungs to really fill up and get much needed oxygen into our cells. Our fast paced, high stress, modern lives have led us to shallow breathing instead of doing what we did as babies. We started out breathing so deep our bellies expanded. What happened along the way that we stopped?

I'm not trying to sell a deep breathing course. I am suggesting you get a singing coach though. Just joking. Sort of. This is where I learned to apply the techniques so you know... What I am trying to do is open up your eyes to the truth about aerobics. Whether you would like to take a martial arts class, or maybe even play golf then that's what you should do! But in the golf example, golf alone won't raise your heart rate enough or supply you with enough oxygen to give you the healthful results you're after. However, having the combination of golf AND something that induces deep breathing will! And hopefully you KEEP deep breathing even when you're NOT exercising….

You weight lift for strength. You perform cardio for endurance. We do both of these things so we continue to enjoy doing 'everyday' things and perhaps to give us the desired results in tone or fat loss. Either way, you are much more apt to make any form of exercise a long term part of your lifestyle if you can do something you enjoy at the SAME TIME. So what does all this mean to you? Well, I'm hoping that you realize that you don't have to seek high tech equipment or expensive memberships to achieve your health goals.

You can join a martial arts class or find something similar you can do right in your own home! It takes a whole lot less time and money than what you think and I bet my bottom dollar that it can be a whole lot more fun than you expect! The funny thing is, now that I practice this, I have cut to 15 minutes instead of 3 times that and I am much leaner, healthier, fuller, and stronger than ever before. I am not kidding when I say I am in better shape and carry less fat than when I weighed 50 pounds lighter. It's amazing. And I am the benefits roll over into all areas of my life. Sure, you may be a lady looking to lose maybe 10, 20 or 50 pounds instead of gaining muscle. But it's all relative. Although you need aerobic exercise to strengthen your heart, lungs, and veins in order to pump nutrients to your muscles and toxins out of your system, it is still NOT the best way to lose body fat. No matter what you believe or how you think that others you admire train, I am here to tell you that you must first diet right, and then second, weight lift with a brief but intense bout of cardio after each session if you want to look your best. This limited amount of aerobics is enough to increase your vital capacity (the useable portion of your lungs) if you really do give it your all.

The problem is, most people do not know how hard is hard enough to achieve visible results. The experts say you know you are working hard enough if you use the figure found by deducting your age from 220 and multiplying that by .7 (it determines the heart rate in beats per minute required for proper cardiovascular work). If you are 30, it doesn't matter if you weigh 100 or 800 pounds, you will deduct 30 from 220 which is 190 and multiplying that by .7 and get 133. So if you are any-where around 133 beats a minute, you're 'in the zone' for fat loss. But what if you are 90 years old? Well, 220 - 90 = 130 x .7 = 90 beats a minute maximum...

I say just get off your butt, weight train for 20 minutes, check and see if this doesn't double your resting heart rate. If not, that's alright, see if you are at least working hard enough to breath heavy without gasping for air. If so, great, if not, then aerobics are not going to help you burn fat.

After 15 minutes of, as I like to say, "Huff and Puff", leave. You're done. And the best aerobic machines to use for this are recumbent cycles and rowing machines in my opinion. Ladies, stair masters do work your butt, however they also lead to large calves (unattractive) and so does walking on a treadmill at an incline (or walking too fast without actually jogging). Keep in mind, as time progresses and weeks pass, you will be able to increase the intensity of your aerobic exercise (by walking faster, rowing faster, riding faster), but once you can jog, either move to another exercise or start jogging. In other words, you must strive to 'travel' further in the same time frame, every ses-sion, if you want to keep burning fat.

What if you're 90? What if you have high blood pressure? F.Y.I. The American Heart Association says blood pressure above 140mm Hg systolic and 90mm Hg diastolic is high and 120 'over' 70 is what's considered healthy. Systolic is the amount of pressure against your artery walls during the heart's contraction and diastolic is the pressure or ease thereof during the heart's relaxation period between beats. Aerobics will elevate your blood pressure a bit but this is safe because it's under limited and controlled durations.

Think of it as doing something to open up clogged drains and allowing for clearer 'breathing' passages while at rest. The research to confirm this was performed by testing the four measures of cardiovascular health in both athletic clientele and seniors. The areas studied were heart rate, maximum oxygen uptake, stroke volume, and ejection fraction. The most enhanced individual progress reported clinically came from short bursts of exercise, not continual aerobic movement. What does this mean? Ever lost your breath after only a few sets of weights? That was your aerobic pathway taking over after the an-aerobic pathway (weight lifting) ended.

Your body started building its cardiovascularity without you actually doing anything 'aerobic'. Go figure. Notice what happens the next time you lift a weight or start breathing heavy during a martial arts class or carrying groceries. It's all the same. Do you understand what I am getting at? You do not need a lot of aerobics in your life to make progress. What type of aerobics you choose should be selected based upon what will allow you to perform greater intensity from session to session and also allows for enough variety you can keep from being bored. What do I do?

Sometimes I run. Sometimes I do sprints. Sometimes I ride a bike. But twice a week I practice martial arts of course. Some of you think I mean that I take Tae Bo or use video cassettes. No, that's not it. Remember what I do for a living? I own a martial arts studio. So for 15 minutes after I am depleted from lifting weights, I hit the heavy bag, kick it or grapple with a stronger student. If Billy Blanks got you off your butt and his tapes are what motivated you to exercise, God bless him. But if you do his or any other form of cardio for more than 20 minutes until you're dropped your fat down, you are defeating the purpose. Look at all the fat aerobic instructors and women who never lose a pound if you do not believe me.

Too much cardio eats away at your muscle. Not eating right doesn't make matters better. In fact, if you limit your cardio to 15 minutes after weights, I honestly feel you can add a few sessions on the side at 20 minutes each every week and be just fine. I do not encourage this at first because I believe you will misunderstand what that means and abuse the privilege, but I think you understand. It is alright to do 2 or 3 sessions of aerobics a week extra if you do not exceed 20 minutes a session, if you have a protein meal before hand, and if you are at least down to those last 10 to 15 pounds of fat to burn.

I have already mentioned this. Until then, stick to the rules, please. You really do not need more. Unless your heart rate is up to 50% of your max heart rate (which is also achieved through weight training) and you have depleted your glycogen (muscle energy) levels without losing muscle (through weight training too) aerobics are not going to help you burn anyhow. Remember when you first started running or riding a bike? You only went so far for the longest time, like a mile at the most, but one day, ONE DAY, out of nowhere, you decided to keep going and actually was able to keep going further than expected? Say for 6 or 10 or maybe more miles?

What gives? You didn't train for that. You only trained for a mile at a shot. All you need is a little conditioning to be capable of a lot of activity believe it or not. Aerobics only do 'so much' for you. Weight training does the rest. If we train hard for short bursts, the conditioning will allow for longer ones almost automatically. And again, I like Billy Blanks. He is motivating. I like Bruce Lee too. But I do not pretend martial arts aerobics will make me into a martial artist nor allow me to understand what it is like to defend myself if necessary. Many classes I have taken in the past were classes of just kicks, punches, combinations, abdominal exercises and maybe some other stuff.

It can be grueling and tiring. Problem is, I remember many students not getting into better shape taking the classes and others that just couldn't last a full hour long session. We know that was partially due to their not eating right and weight training. But like myself, at one point, it was also due to doing too much aerobic oriented work. Being able to last an hour long of aerobics doesn't necessarily mean you are better conditioned. I know plenty of marathon runners that spend 9 months of the year sick as dogs. Nor do aerobics teach you to defend yourselves.

A lot of ladies take Tae Bo and some of you have bought the videos thinking what you learn will protect you from a purse snatcher or allow you to stand up for your lady in a bar. Not true. Yes, I want you to look at martial arts as aerobic, but I do not want you to look at aerobics as martial arts. It is my intention to help those of you who want variety in your aerobics to think of yourselves as potential students of the martial arts. Through just a little training, 15 minutes, 3 days a week, maybe even only 2, we can teach you how to sharpen and hone the natural tools you didn't even know you had. This is important because like it or not, odds are, all of us at one time or another will be attacked.

Through just 15 minutes of work after each weight training session spent either with a partner or a punching bag, you may be more than able to walk away from that attack standing tall. No one wants to mess with someone who at least knows one or two moves to defend themselves. They haven't a clue what else is in your arsenal, so most often, they back off rather than push the issue. You do not have to look like Arnold, nor have the skills of Jackie Chan. But you should be able to get through a weight training session and then 12 minutes of punches and kicks without getting too winded if you expect to protect yourself.

No attack will ever last 40 minutes, so brief and quick is key here. If you can make it through a training session that's 30 minutes total, you can make it through a purse snatcher or drunken buffoon attack. To accomplish this, you must practice techniques that you have seen work or are proven to be the most beneficial. Once you have studied and rehearsed them to a point they are easy, learn others. I also recommend getting instruction in boxing. Learn to use a speed bag. There is nothing like hitting the speed bag after a workout.

Besides, your opponent may be an out of work boxer. You do not necessarily need to know ring strategy, but learning how to use your hands for a real fighting situation may come important. Knocking a bag around like Rocky Balboa can be quite cardio-vascular. You'll see once you try it. Kicking and punching the air is not true preparation for self defense. You need to actually strike something or have a friend to beat on (just kidding, don't try to hurt someone). If you are looking into getting a heavy bag for your home to practice with, get one that hangs low around your shin level and yet is tall enough that it's around 6 foot high.

Eventually you will move up to rehearsing knee and shin blows. Hey, an opponent on the street may be a pro at kickboxing! I do not want you paranoid that you're being stalked or there is always a chance you may be attacked, but that is how people get hurt. They aren't prepared if they are. My next suggestion here is that you look into ground fighting, grappling, wrestling or Gracie Barra Jiu Jitsu. It will come as quite a surprise as to how much fat you will lose learning to go one on one with an attacker, how confident you will become in your everyday life and how much you will learn to respect others by learning and rehearsing these arts 15 minutes, 3 times a week. Do not become fascinated by belts and competitions.

On the street, there isn't time to find out what rank the opponent is nor see if the referee is watching to keep them from getting too rough. Your self-protection rests in your own hands. There are a thousand different moves and techniques and a million different ways of applying them. Every situation and instructor is going to be different. The moves or techniques that you use against a short fighter, may not work against a taller fighter, or a thinner opponent as it would a fatter, men vs. women and vice versa.

Your instructor will teach you what they feel is most beneficial but you may let them know you really are looking for something specific. No matter the situation, you must always consider the possibility that a trip to the store, to the gym, the bank or worse, sleeping at home, may lead to an attack by a stranger or someone we previously trusted. It is better to be prepared and not have to use your skills, rather than to need skills and not have any! Here are a few things to keep in mind when training to defend yourself:

Keep your eyes open and pay attention to your opponent's moves. Attack directly, strike as though you will only need to strike once but follow through with as many more blows as necessary. That will either give the attacker second thoughts or you're gonna successfully stop them! Besides that, know the ground, the area, and even the direction of the sun and wind around you. I wouldn't throw kicks on a wet surface. I wouldn't stand with my face in the wind or sun because it's blinding. Circle the opponent to let the wind blow or sun shine on them instead. Got a good idea of what you need to do now?

Ladies, try this. It will benefit you. Besides, stair masters do not work your butt, they lead to large calves (unattractive) and so does walking on an incline (or walking too fast) on a treadmill. Speaking of which, if you are able to increase the intensity of the exercise (by walking faster, rowing faster, riding faster) you better if you want to keep burning fat, but the hard core 10 to 15 minute duration rule must never be exceeded. Your body will start burning the glucose stored as glycogen (body starch) in your muscles and liver if you do. If I taught you today that you need only short aerobic training to get results, that variety is OK and that learning to defend yourself not only makes sense but it can be substituted for cardio work a few times a week, then my job is done.

For more on martial arts. See Don Lemmon's
www.martialartschampions.com

MY QVC EXERCISE VIDEO PROJECT

What a year this was. Get ready for some fur to fly. I will be subtle but I haven't a lot of good things to say here today. It began in late May, early June of 1996. 15 months later it was practically done. 18 months later completely done. I had toyed with the idea of exercise videos to show my clients what I expected of them prior to taking them to the gym myself. But then when the video business took off, I wanted to take it up another notch. At first, I recruited 50 friends and clients who would each perform one exercise apiece under my instruction. But the cost of producing a video and having it edited in Vegas was a joke at the time.

The quality produced for the price they demanded was unfounded. To get the quality I wanted… Forget about it. I may as well have been filming a feature film. So in June, I headed east. Pittsburgh that is. Why Pittsburgh? The plan was to get these videos on television to put a halt on Tony Little and Susan Powter's domination over people who really didn't know any better. QVC is just outside of Philadelphia. Pittsburgh is just outside of Youngstown, near where I grew up. I made a few calls and got a hold of the illustrious photographer JM Manion because he managed a few of the girls I was working with.

In July, he introduced me to Johnny Albert, who runs the NPC Clothing Warehouse and films video on the side. Since he seemed to know what he was doing, had a decent track record and quoted a price that seemed to make sense to me, I relocated from Vegas to Ohio officially, once and for all it seemed, in August.

By September, I had that much ready and booked the various flights to have my 'stars' flown in to film. I also had former Danger Danger vocalist Ted Poley and Tommy Lee guitarist J3 slated to handle most of the soundtrack for me. We first filmed one day near the middle of October, 1996 from around 6:30 p.m. to 2:00 a.m. in the morning.

It was a tough day because everyone flew in just that day to film this for me. Some to Cleveland, some to Pittsburgh, a couple from Vegas, a couple from Florida, another from Baltimore and right from the start, things were off schedule. We didn't have time to spare because half of them planned to also leave that same night. The first glitch involved having one car go to Cleveland and another to Pittsburgh at the same time to pick up two groups of people from two separate airports then meeting in the middle of both cities for lunch.

Once we all co-ordinated in Youngstown (the middle ground), a third of the people never showed. And due to even worse planning, we had to drive all the way back to Pittsburgh again to film. After tracking down the third party (who couldn't leave without an extra 45 minutes on makeup), we finally made it back to town and were all ready and made up for the shoot. Trouble was, the 5 p.m. shooting didn't start until 6:30! I cannot begin to explain how stressful this day was. And to top it off, we were filming this thing in the private gym of the man who basically runs American bodybuilding these days, Jim Manion.

The initial problem once we arrived on set was that some of my 'stars' thought they were in a candy store. The gym attaches to the NPC Clothing Warehouse. The NPC corp carries a popular line of workout clothing. I didn't know about this until afterward, but half the cast stole several hundred dollars in clothing that day. Besides that, the rest of the shoot was fun. I suppose...

The thing that wasn't fun was the effect of all this stress on my health. I was 'advised' by my image consultants, legal reps and everyone else to drop my weight down to 180 pounds from 210 without becoming too muscular in the process for the shoot. They felt I would appeal better to 'middle America' than a bloated Tony Little or feminist Susan Powter could that way. I personally felt horrible and looked malnourished. I am not saying this because I am vain.

I am saying my true body weight is 200 to 205 not 180. The weight loss triggered a loss of immunity which allowed a cold to linger the entire month. On top of it, I had to force myself to work straight through it all. They also made me get a short haircut for the first time in Lord knows how long. Someone want to send me a Badge of Honor? Sniffle, sniffle. I couldn't win either way but I did whatever I needed to in order to get this thing on television, with the exception of wearing nylons, screaming, dancing, sweating, perming my hair or showing off my butt sitting next to an obese woman crying like Richard Simmons. Hey, I am just telling you like it is, that's all.

The concept for the video was nothing more than having some very interesting people seen exercising with me coaching them a little, but I never planned on doing my own narrative. I wanted to maintain a hint of mystery to it all. A sort of 'Who is this Don Lemmon character?' approach. I am sure the people who eventually saw it, appreciated it for what it was worth. However, despite explaining this concept to Johnny, the day of the shoot he went for something different. He wanted me to explain to him why we were doing the exercises differently than he was used to. I thought he 'knew' or should have known that wasn't the plan, but he forgot. After that hurdle was crossed, we were home free. Well, except for the one girl missing her flight due to these delays and mishaps…

The people filming with me that day were the ultra ripped big tan man, Mr. America, Lee Apperson who just came back from his Mr. Universe contest. Las Vegas showgirl "Angela" (whom we later found out was a stripper) and Angela's boyfriend martial artist, Matthew Richard Pollino. Both were dead tired from their constant bickering, overnight flights…

Neither of the latter performed on film well enough that we could use much of their footage. I was a bit let down by that. I have a funny side note about Lee Apperson who weighed 245 pounds the day of the shoot and Matt who calls himself TIGER. "Tiger" wouldn't tell Lee his real name and age so Lee challenged him to a brawl over it. It was funny when he was 21, 10 years ago but now that he is 30, it's plain silly. His name is Matthew Pollino and before moving from L.A. he ripped me off for a lot of money. Pat the guy on the back for being such a class act if you see him. The blonde lady I used, reigning fitness queen, Theresa Hessler, a legal assistant living with a stripper boyfriend too at the time, showed up in the best shape of the girls we shot. She is recently divorced from a bodybuilder I think.

If you run into her, ask her about the time we all went out, she got drunk and then left me stranded at the nite club, not cool. We also used my chiropractor at that shoot. He only trained with me a few times prior to the shoot to get used to the work-out but for someone who was supposedly a former NFL prospect, he sure whined and complained a lot! Just kidding pal, and no, the lack of a tan wasn't a problem! We got all the tan we needed from Florida's own buff chick, National bodybuild-ing champ, Michelle Ralabate. A gymnast, who I also think has piercing everywhere on her body, later worked at a couple of conventions with me and is quite the crowd favorite.

Those were the six people we filmed that day. At around 3:30 a.m. I finally hit the hay but had to get up, pick up Lee from the hotel, drop him off at the airport, drive back to Pittsburgh, get Michelle, take her to another airport and after that, go see Matt and Angela for a bit before we took them to the airport. Funny I say that because we had such a headache with that girl we actually drove them to the airport and dropped them off without caring what flight they took. Pretty sad, isn't it?

What I was beginning to learn was that people who get into

professions that depend on their looks, body or boobs, tend to have quite a few issues. And I was a babysitter. When you drop a bunch of these people off in the same room, you either have a lot of fake behavior, two-faced discussions or cat fighting. I know it sounds like that's what I am doing right now myself but it's not. I just want you to know, this isn't exactly what you think it is… That following weekend we all flew to Dallas for a fitness convention where we debuted the raw footage. The quality of the filming was great. It wasn't edited so it was obvious that half of Matt and Angela's scenes needed redone.

As soon as I got back to Ohio, I cast the guy you see in the video with a crew cut, Mr. USA Danny Weigand and the alluring red head with an amazing smile from the Ms Galaxy, Janie Tomasovich. These two were the easiest to work with and I haven't a single complaint whatsoever about them, however, there is a great out take from the second video where Janie makes it clear she wants nowhere near a couple of the other fitness models we used! That was a HILARIOUS moment!

The people I used ranged from 4'11" tall to 6'3". They weighed from 100 to 250 pounds and each came in varying degrees of physical conditioning. Only 2 of them were 'ripped' or really low in body fat. I used a variety of people and physiques to show that all goals can be met using the same exercise routines. I wish things had gone a little better and these videos went on the market as planned because even today, they really aren't bad at all. The first hitch in getting them done occurred in December after expecting the videos to be ready by Christmas. They weren't. In fact, it wasn't until January that the actual intro was brought to me. I wasn't happy. I had put down several thousand dollars on the editing and all I had was a 3 minute introduction.

The funny thing is that the footage we have isn't even out dated today with the exception that no one in them is still performing. In January while waiting for the final cut I signed on an old friend from Chippendales, Bernie Tavis and David Lee Roth's guitarist supplied some more soundtrack bytes for the defunct project. Las Vegan Jeff McMullens played the riffs between segments. Narration was handled by Youngstown Ohio's award winning morning radio hosts, AC McCullough and Kelly Stevens. Too bad it was never edited properly and completed. The 43 minute tape it became is nonetheless entertaining.

Despite the glitches here and there, home styled guerilla editing, having a large crew and a lot of guests on the set getting in the way, I am proud to say, there is a lot of cool stuff captured. If you listen closely to the advice given in the second two shoots especially, it is cleverly geared towards not only the beginner but also the seasoned pro. This product could have been a gem if completed.

By late March 1997 I had gained 20 pounds back and was feeling 100% better. That's when I planned the next two videos. You will note the difference between the various workout segments, and footage from October, 1996 to May, 1997 at the second video shoot of my condition and health too. The May shoot was actually two shoots sandwiched between two conventions. The first in Pittsburgh at the same gym and the second in Youngstown at the gym I leased my office in.

I have of course included a number of behind the scenes shots from this stuff too. Watching it again shows how silly we are. I had a good time during this shoot. There wasn't as much rushing around and I think it shows. We did have a problem with one of the girls thinking she was better than everyone else and demanding preferential treatment. Tell me you cannot pick which one it was when you see this! Another night, the night before the filming, we spent all our time out chasing down a stolen car! We had to get the local authorities AND the FBI involved. The guy who caused the trouble stole one of the girl's wallets too.

Also in the video shoot this time besides, Janie and Matt again, are Mr. Austria Markus Daxl, martial artist Artie Kaikou, Hawaiian fitness queen Dale Tomita, masters champ Jesse Mathesen benching 405 lbs, Ms World Karen Hulse stretching out, Ms Olympia Carol Semple showing us her new braces and of course, Johnny behind the lens. We shot noon to midnight. AGAIN. "We shoot til we finish or til we drop." This particular video was geared more towards the bodybuilder or fitness competitor but the exercises are those folks at any level can enjoy. Everyone there was in great shape. No complaints except that everyone again seemed to think they were more important than anyone else with the exception of a couple. I won't say who.

A week later we planned to shoot in the gym where I was renting space for my offices back in Youngstown, Ohio. Just a week after filming the second video, I have to admit, I was a little burnt out. This video featured buff World Toughman Champ Ray Hammond benching 500, Ms Fitness Ohio Michelle Talboo, Artie Kaikou again, who is shown teaching a martial arts class.

The kids in one out take deservingly attack and beat me up as Ms International Susie Curry rehearses her fitness routine. There is more footage of the crew taking a Spinning class with Ray. My brother, and my mother even make cameos (very funny, I caught them eating all the sponsor's foods), model Brian Blazek, Theresa Hessler again (never again) and the always charming Danny Weigand once more. We were set for a good time… There was a room full of my local clients at the time and toasts of wine all around. Yes, if you watch closely, that's me having a beer with Pan Am games tae kwon do medallist Angela Wolbert and Susie Curry during a break in front of a BALANCE Nutrition snack bars sign.

They endorsed the shoot before the company was bought by Hershey. I no longer eat their bars to say the least. There is plenty of my sarcastic wit exchanged between most of the guests on this tape. It's worth watching just to see how crazy we can be. Were we drunk? Not at all. At least I wasn't. I do not condone drinking and working out at the same time. Who bought it then? See the video and the guilty party will be more than obvious. The devil is a woman in a white sports bra. The next day after the shoot, we hung out at the Mr Ohio show I sponsored. I had a dozen people there and the video stars handed out the trophies. Was another good time.

Again, you must see the footage to believe it! If you listen to our discussions throughout this tape in particular, some of the info you get you couldn't pay any trainer on earth for. Ms North America Erica Kern, who is also on this 3rd video did not come to shoot her segments until June. During the next couple of months while I was still waiting for my first video to get edited, we began formulating the KNOW HOW Food products. In August (still waiting) I did a morning television show where we debuted my own line of surgically pure bottled water, the original video box covers, the original book cover too. Some of the supplements like my coffee replacements and healthy snow cone machines were partly my concept to trick people into not making themselves sick by using the junk food versions of these items. It caused quite a National stir that caught me by surprise. I spent most of the interview shutting down the reporter.

Let's not forget something else about these videos. I also covered stretching like no one else has still ever done to date. I know you may be thinking a bench is a bench, a stretch is a stretch but that is NOT true. I preview all the stretching techniques my clients are taught one on one here. You know what bothered me the most about the shoots? Not that the footage wasn't exactly what I wanted but that the little things the cameraman or editor could have fixed, they didn't.

Besides editing issues that were never resolved, being billed triple what was originally discussed, charged for fixing mistakes that turned into more mistakes, some of the athletes had managers, agents or sponsors that said they couldn't continue to endorse me unless I began paying them. This obviously set distribution back even further (to present day). I suffered a financial loss that took until 2001 to settle. I refused to release these videos in any way, shape or form but here we are. I have decided to do it anyhow.

The thing is, while this whole project has left a sick feeling in my stomach, can you imagine being so far ahead of your time, that no one is still, to this day, even remotely close to catching up with your ideas? Well, top it off by just 'sitting' on such footage. I am tired of sitting.

I have finally put together some of the stuff using the 'stars' who pulled through in 1996 and 1997 and am offering it unedited for the first time ever via my website. We actually have 5 total workouts on the original video, 18 more complete unedited workouts with the various personalities performing them digitized in rough form, ready for you now. They are burned to a CD and are in Windows Media format.

So, for the first time, here we go… Since you have read the book so far you understand why you cannot do more than what I suggest here and that only one set to failure or one set with more weight or more reps than your previous effort is all you need. Any workouts with more than 10 total sets include extra movements that are nothing more than warmups, light movements or something to get the blood going in cold weather. No more than 10 sets a workout are performed to failure and no more than 20 total sets are ever performed (important, remember, half are warm-ups). Workouts #3 through #20 are on the "Official Know How RAW Exercise Video Footage From The 1997 QVC Project" CD. Workouts #1, #2 and #26 will be available in 2003 and Workouts #21 through #25 are part of the still unreleased 40 or so minute long video. Here are what each workout features. Enjoy...

WORKOUT #1 (3 exercises) - Taken from the book, not on video YET...
Exercises are: military press, bent over row, leg press

WORKOUT #2 (3 exercises) - Taken from the book, not on video YET...
Exercises are: Squat, pulldown, bench press

VIDEO WORKOUT #3 (5 exercises) - featuring Janie Tomasovich

VIDEO WORKOUT #4 (6 exercises) - featuring Markus Daxl and Carol Semple

VIDEO WORKOUT #5 (7 exercises) - featuring Matt Pollino

VIDEO WORKOUT #6 (7 exercises) - featuring The Mathesens

VIDEO WORKOUT #7 (8 exercises) - featuring Angela Wolbert Clark

VIDEO WORKOUT #8 (9 exercises) - featuring Michelle Talboo

VIDEO WORKOUT #9 (9 exercises) - featuring Brian Blazek

VIDEO WORKOUT #10 (10 exercises) - featuring Artie Kaikou

VIDEO WORKOUT #11 (11 exercises) - featuring Momir Sornaz

VIDEO WORKOUT #12 (11 exercises) - featuring Theresa Hessler

VIDEO WORKOUT #13 (11 exercises) - featuring Matt Pollino

VIDEO WORKOUT #14 (12 exercises) - featuring Susie Curry

VIDEO WORKOUT #15 (12 exercises) - featuring Dale Tomita

VIDEO WORKOUT #16 (12 exercises) - featuring Eric Bergman

VIDEO WORKOUT #17 (12 exercises) - featuring Karen Hulse

VIDEO WORKOUT #18 (13 exercises) - featuring Danny Weigand

VIDEO WORKOUT #19 (15 exercises) - featuring Ray Hammond

VIDEO WORKOUT #20 (20 exercises) - featuring Ericca Kern

VIDEO WORKOUTS #21 - 25 From The Initial Original Don Lemmon QVC Video COMING SOON

VIDEO WORKOUT #26 - BONUS ADVANCED SESSION ALSO COMING SOON

Ok, now if you do each of the 26 routines for 2 weeks each, 3 times one week, 2 times the next, then you've got yourself a full year's worth of workouts to go by… If a copy of any of these workouts didn't come with this book, drop by my website at www.freeexercisevideos.com for more info. All 5 hours and 18 workouts on the main video is only $30. The others are $10 each and all include a PDF file to explain the routines. I have other videos we shot available here too.

SELECTING A HOME GYM

I know that most of you believe in me and I have your trust. However, there are others who may read this and feel differently due to the point I want to get across. If this is you, I want to take this moment to help you clearly understand that I will not try to force you or anyone else to follow my advice nor any other program for that matter. It makes no difference to me whether what you think is right is actually 'right' or wrong. I will however attempt to pass along to you what I know in a sincere effort to let the facts be known regardless. So let me explain why this chapter is so important.

There are 4 types of fitness equipment or resistance used to choose from when creating a new routine or setting up a workout that suits your needs. The first is constant resistance exercise equipment. This is the type of stuff where throughout the entire movement, the weight seems to remain the same (you'll understand what this means in a second). The second is variable resistance technology. This is the type of equipment where the resistance or feel of the weight seems to change at some points (like with Nautilus equipment where it gets harder to lift the weight the closer to the muscular contraction point you get). The third type of resistance is static, or isometric exercise. This is the type of movement where there is no actual movement up or down at all with the exception of the pushing or pulling effect itself you use to cause the muscle to contract. Last but not least we have accommodating resistance. This form of exercise is the type where both the weight and the speed are easily controlled by the lifter.

You cannot perform them all at once, nor should you try to, especially all in one session. You probably don't have access to all the different machine types to do so even if you wanted to. Despite machines being easier and safer to use that barbells and dumb bells in most cases, you cannot forgo free style weights for the machines. While machines isolate your muscles better than barbells or dumbbells, without barbells, you are never going to fully develop your co-ordination skills, strength nor burn the fat you want to. Why? Because you need to use all different forms of resistance and no routine is good unless it is first run it's course and then restructured for variety.

If you really want to reach your full potential, you will use a little of anything and everything you can get your hands on to train with. Where do you begin? Just pick one. If I had to pick, I would probably select a different technology depending the muscle. Each muscle reacts better or best depending on what one we are discussing. I might say that something like the original Nautilus machines with their variable resistances. If I hadn't much of a choice, ANYTHING WILL DO. Just lift something!

Have you seen any of those fitness infomercials on late night television? The ones where all you need is to make three easy payments and you will soon have the perfect body of your dreams using their wonderful toys. If that's true, then why don't you or anyone else have the body of their dreams using this junk? And why do only washed up TV stars, not current or movie stars, hawk that crap? Career INTEGRITY. Keep in mind, no matter who is endorsing those products on TV, anything that works only one muscle or offers little resistance, isn't worth wasting your time on. In fact, the woman who supposedly developed the first abdominal curler or cruncher (or whatever it was) ever sold on modern TV bragged to us one day that her product was pure junk and that she never even used it. She was a member of my gym at the time QVC sold her junk!

Millions of Americans buy home gym equipment every year. I am sure you know someone who has something off TV and does NOT use it! Be it one piece of equipment or many, nothing works unless it offers more than one exercise and one of the top 4 forms of resistance. I realize having a gym membership doesn't guarantee you'll exercise either. Some of us lack the time. And the gyms themselves are not exactly jumping through hoops for you to attend either. They like the club being empty because they can sell more memberships that way. Besides, they already have your cash, monthly credit card or automatic debit payment anyways.

If you aren't wasting the investment, a gym membership is good since you get to use all the different equipment that obviously can't fit in your house but I do not always feel like nor have the opportunity to attend. I am NOT attacking gyms. I travel, I get overloaded with work, and who knows your reasoning? I have a solution to all of this. Go to the gym when you can, say twice a week, then use an affordable, total body home gym on another day or whenever you can't get to the gym. EVEN WHEN YOU TRAVEL. What gym fits in your purse or is no bigger than a folded t-shirts?

You have probably seen the Bodylastics product on QVC alongside the crap I wouldn't touch with a ten foot pole. It is the elastic band home gym kit put together by my good friend Blake Kassel. He is not just the owner of the Bodylastics company and I am not just an endorser, but we are both proud users. And he has become such a good friend of mine that he actually mentioned Don Lemmon's KNOW HOW briefly in his last QVC appearance! If you haven't personally heard of him, that's alright. Grab some water, and check this out. The Bodylastics kit is something similar to the elastic bands used in aerobics classes except these ones have tension equal anywhere from 5 to 100's of pounds in my favorite, VARIABLE resistance! No kidding. This home gym is so innovative that it has been featured in numerous national publications like Glamour, New Woman, Delta Sky, Woman's World, Jane, Men's Exercise, Prevention, You Gotta Read This and Essence magazines.

What at first appears to be nothing more than a simple set of 4 rubber bands with handles is really something that professional athletes, personal trainers and bodybuilders use too. What you have here is a complete barbell set or what's close to a complete fitness center membership all in one 2 pound bag. The only difference is that this gym doesn't have anyone waiting in line ahead of you and you won't need to clear an entire garage out to make room for it. And for less than the cost of one month at any health club, Men, Women, Children, the Elderly, and the Athletic, can all use this anytime, and anywhere. It fits in a suitcase or a purse and all you need is the space around you at arms length to use it. Our friends in Japan, where living spaces are quite limited, really seem to love us for that!

I know that personally, I regret leaving home for business trips because that means I must actually go out and find a gym because hotels rarely have anything worth using and the process is such a pain in the neck. I have spent way too much time looking for the local gyms, calling them one by one for directions, and you know the routine.... Getting ready, driving there, finding parking, signing in, waiting for a guest tour, making my way around the naked people hanging out in the locker room for no apparent reason, finally getting to work out, only to wait in line for the equipment, then trying to get back to the hotel or home again … It's a 4 hour process for a 30 minute workout that I just don't have time for.

I have traveled by car and by plane across the United States so many times I can't even assume to remember how often that I have experienced headaches with owners, people behind the counter thinking they have power for a change or salespeople that really ought to be trying to sell local customers. There is one gym that sticks out in my mind because they treated me like I was a member for years each time I passed through. That gym is called Popeye's and it is located in Topeka, Kansas. I am not kidding when I say that most everywhere else I have been I felt like I was asking people if I could pull their teeth rather than paying them to use their clubs. These days, I do not even bother. I use my Bodylastics kit.

Friends of mine use Bodylastics to warm themselves up before they go on stage, doing a photo shoot, looking pumped up for a date or even heading out on to the playing field to warm up. Imagine how much of a benefit it is not to lug dumbbells around with you everywhere from now on for these things. I like the kit so much I had Blake send me extra straps so I can work up to an amazing 500 pounds of resistance on some of my favorite movements.... Can you picture this? I can take a broom stick, slide it through the handles, place the stick across my back, and suddenly I am squatting hundreds of pounds and there's no weight to rack or unrack afterwards! By simply using any given number of the four different sized elastic bands, the kit accommodates almost all of the various levels of strength you could imagine between a pro wrestler and a grandparent.

I used to be a bodybuilder. My close friends still are or have become pro athletes. None of us could do a complete curl or a squat using the entire four bands for 10 reps on our first attempt. A few of us couldn't do all 4 bands at all on most movements. That's a lot of resistance. And I am a pretty strong guy! Drop a couple bands and seconds later, your father can start to use them. The unique clip system attached to both ends of the bands is what allows you to vary the resistance or weight lifted so quick. And because of the handles, there are so many exercises you can perform with these things. Not only does each muscle group have several choices of exercise, but by varying the number of bands, you can get the maximum stimulus for each without ever feeling under-worked or over-worked at any level you have achieved.

Other elastic sets come with either both handles permanently attached to one elastic (which doesn't allow you to use more than one band), or you are forced to adjust the resistance level by rolling up the rubber. This causes wobbling, a disruption of the body's natural movement and more often than not, slippage and injury. Imagine what happens if the bands unravel. WHAP!

Right in the face! I couldn't let my kid or grand mother use something like that. This is something I believe makes this better than Bowflex and Soloflex combined. Trust me, you don't need bulky equipment to get into shape. You simply need something that adds resistance to your exercise. Something that makes working against gravity a little tougher. The Bodylastics home gym can effectively do all of the above for right around $40.00 You read that right. You are about to not only save hundreds if not thousands of dollars on exercise equipment, but you can even get this product for less than the official Bodylastics website and QVC charges.

It was proven years ago that the only way to change the shape or appearance of your body is to make your muscles tone. The only way to do that is to make them stronger. To gain strength, a muscle must lengthen (eccentric movement) and shorten (concentric contraction) against some form of resistance. But your muscles are blind. They do not know, nor care, if you are curling a barbell, a dumbbell or a machine. They only know that you are working against some sort of resistance and variable resistance is best, but you need something besides a machine to build co-ordination and skill at the same time. As long as this is met and it is something heavy enough for you to feel the stress, this resistance can come in the form of Bodylastics or bricks. It doesn't matter. Bricks unfortunately cannot allow for the following exercises:

Pushups (yes, pushups, but now they can be performed with as much resistance as bench presses), chest flyes (normally done with dumbbells), crossovers (without cables), side lateral shoulder raises (without dumbbells or a machine), front shoulder raises (ditto), front and rear military presses (no barbell needed), lat pull downs (goodbye lat machine), pullovers, bent over rows, seated rows, shrugs, rear pull downs, squats, lunges, hip extensions, leg extensions, deadlifts, hamstring curls, calf raises, biceps curls, preacher curls, overhead triceps extensions, kickbacks, tricep pushdowns, situps, crunches (better than any ab roller), hyperextensions, inclined movements, forearm exercises and MORE... I even figured out how to leg presses with these things.

What's even more important to point out besides variety is the fact you can perform all movements through a complete range of motion. I think I made it clear how vital that is to developing quick and permanent results over the years.

The one concern we have is that you go out and try to over-stretch the elastics. The bands carry an extensive warranty. If they snap, we replace them. But do not think for a second that if it's clear you are playing tug of war with them from across the room or using the bands to strap down furniture on a truck that it won't result in weakening and/or breakage.

So the truth of the matter is that you must decide, is it worth having a kit like this that costs around $40 to replace the gym on the days you haven't access to the club? Yes it is. But then again, maybe you haven't anything to train on at home to begin with and you are considering other options. Whatever equipment interests you, it must still meet the demands of allowing for progression. If you cannot add weight to an exercise when you need to or cannot move up the speed on a cardio machine fast enough to keep up with your conditioning, you're in trouble. Our entire lives are based on trying for more and more. Do not forget this fact. The only other piece of home gym equipment I use is a stationary bike. It cost me a few hundred dollars and it's a bike that's been on the market for over 30 years. I like it.

I do not recommend or endorse any particular brand name or type of equipment unless I like it. I do not know how much space you have to work with so I will leave it at that. As far as health club equipment, I love Med-x, Hammer Strength, Nautilus, barbells, dumbbells and other properly built pieces of equipment that come in all sorts of shapes and sizes. I like aerobic rowing machines and bikes more than I like treadmills and stair climbers. But I haven't room for all of them at home, in fact most of them, and I do not always feel like fighting traffic even locally and that's why I have my little rubber band kit.

However, it's important that you do your own research and choose the items that are best for you. I've provided you with plenty of info to build upon. It's now up to you to gather more information. Check out Blake's site at www.bodylastics.com Tell the Rubber Band Man I sent you so you can save $10. Otherwise, drop me a line or send a check for $40 made out to BODYLASTICS and I will forward it off to him.

CLOSING THOUGHTS

This book summarizes everything I show my clients who come seeking guidance from me their first 90 days on the program (Hmmm… Maybe I should charge more for this book…). I mean really, I could go ahead and charge you, like I charged them, $150 a session for 5 sessions every two weeks all month long for 3 months to learn what I have to offer here or we could wrap it up into a tight package of a few hundred pages for less than 10 minutes on the phone with me. I wonder which will save you the most time and money. What lies inside the pages of this chapter are the mysteries of Willy Wonka's Chocolate Factory.

The first edition of my program was only 28 pages and left a lot of what you were craving hidden from view. It sold 25,000 copies and detailed the exact training programs and dietary routines to achieve what those you emulate have. Imagine, all you need forever in just 28 pages. Nothing else. Thanks to your demand, there is almost 20 times the amount of pages here. It wouldn't have been possible without support. Growth depends upon it.

I want to thank and say that I am forever grateful that God or whomever is up there allowed my time on Earth to overlap with so many amazing people.

Jason Gateman (www.thinkbigdesigns.com), Dave Campbell, Blake Kassel (www.bodylastics.com), Paul Becker, Harold Whiting, Robert Gaffney (www.omeganutrition.com), Dr Gary Eversole (www.drgaryeversoledc.com), Tom Clark, Suzanne Clark and Ron Stuckey (www.tjclarkminerals.com), Gary Augustine Warren (www.chhpresents.com), Harrison Khordestani, Charles Sproule, Dave Grisaffi, David Young, John Balik (www.ironmanmagazine.com), Nadia Alterio (www.nadiaalterio.com) and if you were forgotten, forgive me.

This list is off the top of my head after weeks of nonstop typing and just trying to think of people who have emailed me lately! This book is almost entirely dedicated to my daughter Carly in loving memory to Carly's Grand Father, Donald E. Lemmon Sr. who passed away just days short of Thanksgiving, 1994.

I would also like to thank those featured on my web site and in my exercise videos, plus the others whose testimonials have helped spread the word about my program. You've seen a lot of my friends in the fitness magazines, on pay-per-view, regular television or even the big screen. May God bless those who came before me, paving my way. If by chance I parallel any-thing you have tried before or anyone else's program you have read before, it is strictly by coincidence. If it is not, I will be the first to admit it.

When I originally came up with the idea for Don Lemmon's Know How I was just getting out of the Army in 1988. That November I spent about two weeks driving up and down the East coast trying to figure out what I was going to do with my life and this book is one of the goals I set for myself. Sure, it's been fun, it looks like a huge success, and I am quite happy, but it hasn't been all smooth sailing. I began working with people one on one for the first time getting paid for it in Fayetteville, North Carolina back in 1988. It immediately became my passion. I am not sure where along the way I can say I fully honed my craft because I have always taught things no one else would. I do know that I feel I am learning something new daily and I sometimes cannot believe I now counsel people from around the World.

Since 1988, I've seen and heard it all. My transcripts have been stolen, sold, quoted and passed about illegally. I have had my articles put in magazines without credit, made and lost friends, seen business associates and (surprise) even family members come and go. It's been heart breaking, but enlightening nonetheless. You see, I have always believed in myself. At times I wanted to give up because everyone around me it seemed either wanted a piece of me they didn't deserve or they tried to keep me from moving forward, but deep inside, I always knew I shouldn't.

I am, always was and will be the Know How forever more. I have lived it, breathed it, walked it, and felt that it just HAD to be brought public ever since pen went to paper. I didn't mean for it to stir so much water along its merry way that the people around me became divided, but it did. The only way to get things done, no matter how long it takes, or how hard it is to accomplish, is to JUST DO THEM FOR YOURSELF, not any-one else. And that's how most of this was accomplished. All alone, with little to no support. Sure, there are a few from start to finish that remained and there are plenty who have jumped on the coat tails since, but where we have come since the begin-nings of it all has been nothing short of inspirational. Point is, you gotta 'keep on keeping on' sometimes.

Not everybody can relate to having a drive so strong or dreams so big that you want to reach the entire World but some of you do. You're the ones who understand. Lord willing, I might just achieve the remainder of my dreams and goals. Speaking of the Lord, I have mentioned previously it is to each their own what they believe in spiritually. I am not suggesting that you change your religion for me and I know you are not interested in changing mine to join yours.

It is just as easy to assume man created a sort of positive belief system to attain power over others, but I believe it is a little more rooted than that. And as long as you and I believe there is good and there is evil, possibly that there is right and there is wrong, and that we both recognize what it is, then we really shouldn't have a problem with one another. Maybe you feel it is others around you that hold you back. Maybe these people need to know in a positive way how you feel about them. If you care about them, let them know. Sometimes people irritate you because it's the only way they know to evoke emotion from you.

Sometimes you simply need to get out of the way of that moving bus. Other times, you are probably the one causing the problems by not opening up. Do your part. Leave it up to the other person after that. I have allowed others to stand in my way over these beliefs at times but I have always maintained my one faith in good versus evil. My strengths are all individual and I believe the reason no one around us shares the same strengths are because we are supposed to help others with what we possess. Even as a child, you knew there was something special about you.

I do not feel I was sent from the heavens but I do feel my strengths were predestined to be within me and that I was meant to be a teacher. I just wanted to take advantage of this moment to say I also do not judge you. So do not judge me. But if up until today you have been struggling to make some spiritual changes that have been put off because you were afraid of what people would think, don't worry about it anymore. Learn more about the foundation of your religion. Not somebody else's interpretation, but the Almighty's, whomever that may be. You have your beliefs coming into this and I have mine. That wasn't part of your decision making process. Do not let it be now. The message I got was that you may be ridiculed, persecuted or crucified for doing what you know is 'right' in this age.

But if you stick to your guns, no matter what, you will receive just reward when your soul moves on after an earthly demise. You may find cows sacred. Maybe even jewelry or cosmetics or bodybuilders are your gods. I am not looking to offend anyone. I just want you to accept me as I accept you. Be positive about this at all times. Discard those around you who aren't positive. Never walk in front of moving busses. Do not take wooden nickels. And realize different cultures are different. I am American.

We use slang you do not. We have religions you do not. We have upbringings you do not. This isn't bad, but it explains our differences. The truth lies within these words. Even if you think I am being sillier than ever right now, you still know the difference between right and wrong. You know you do. As a child, you knew. You chose to rebel or be accepting of that fact as far back as when you were in diapers. Watch a child when they first start to walk and get mischievous.

Everything you do in life revolves around making choices. I have studied theology for years. Most religions offer the same advice. Yes, in America most people use the Bible as a foundation. Sure, it has been revised, edited, etc since it first became available but the storylines haven't changed. It has more in it than you realize. If you are willing to read others, just give this one a shot too. I am not a Bible thumping zealot, I just want us to get to know each other better. In this day and age, too many American religions issue you a Bible but it never gets read. Too many religions come to America and criticize us without knowing what they are talking about. I know, I know, maybe you went to Catholic school or church every Sunday and you already 'know' what's in the Bible.

If it offends you that I say this, that's something within yourself you should take some time to deal with. I also think you should read other religious texts, writings, etc from all around the world so we can better understand those who come here as well. DO THIS. Smile. Laugh. Enjoy. It is in you. Change your bad habits into good habits and lead by example instead of following the same old crowd from now on. Your life tomorrow is based upon whatever decision you make next. The truth lies within these words SO REMEMBER:

1. If what you're doing now is working, KEEP doing it. Don't be silly. Go, Go, Go!

2. If what you're doing now is NOT working, STOP doing it. Face reality. It doesn't work.

3. If you don't know what to do, DON'T do a thing. You may make things worse. Re-read this book.

Be GOOD. Do GOOD. And if anyone ever stands in your way, walk AROUND them NOT over them. Your physique, energy levels, spirituality and newfound health depend upon the commitment you have made today to listen to genuinely basic and common sense things I have presented. I know that when you walk into a law office you expect the people there to know law. When you go to a bar you expect the bartender to know his liquors.

You even depend upon mechanics to know their jobs well enough to work on pretty much anything with a motor in it but things couldn't possibly be further from the truth. People in all professions specialize in particular branches of their field. If your goal is to be taken prisoner by Xena the Warrior Princess or to go on a Legendary Journey with Hercules, I can't help you there. If your goal is to look your best naturally, become healthier doing and enjoy the path for a change, hey, I am your man.

But you'll be surprised at how many people work in this industry that haven't a clue how to teach you these simple things. The path I took is a bit different than you have followed before, but it works, and this is why we are often referred to as The "UN" Diet! If you ever have questions, EMAIL ME:

donlemmon@yougottareadthis.com

You will always have valid concerns and questions. There are many things to take into consideration while making a lifelong commitment to yourself, but I have covered most of them before and to me it is second hand knowledge. I want to see your current diet and training program. No time has ever been more right than now. Especially since NO FRIEND, NO

NEIGHBOR, NO EQUIPMENT, NO GYM in the World GUARANTEES that you will achieve your health and fitness goals by using their services. BUT I DO! I am confident that I can do for you what I have already done for thousands of others. Right now you are probably thinking "Does this guy want me to make an expensive commitment to personal training or phone consultations or something?" NO! It's just the opposite. I want you to email me for FREE!

That's FREE for 30 days if you have the book, FREE each month you get the supplements and FREE on the 90 Day KNOW HOW Plan. Let me make one more thing clear, it is I, Don Lemmon, who will be answering your questions. Not some punk off the street answering phones for minimum wage. However, show a little respect when you contact me. We all can be easily confused or do things we think are right, but aren't, and that leads to frustration. If this happens, understand, it isn't me who is doing whatever you are doing wrong. It is ME though who WILL help you sort it back out and motivate you. So let's work together, not separately on this.

Think of how the lack of motivation to do something held you back and how depression has overwhelmed you without hope until you read this book. All you are doing is seeking help, just like you did when you purchased this program. Well, you've got it. I know you want to enhance your self-esteem, reduce the risk of illness or injury, sleep better, perform your best, look your best, be a better lover and all that. I know you want to get rid of the stress in your life. I will help you via email. Just ask.

I am so insistent on this because there are far too many people who are getting ROBBED at their gyms or health food stores by clowns who get paid $5.75 an hour for part-time work that started as a hobby but turned into a means by which to make a living! Plus, I take YOUR SUCCESS very seriously. If you fail, I do not get your referrals. And I need referrals to keep this business running. If this business fails, I cannot help you nor anyone else ever again. I want to know what time you sleep, wake up, eat, what the foods are and what measures of those foods you ingest happened to be.

Telling me you had a turkey sandwich isn't enough. I want to know how much meat, veggies and bread were there. Do you drink milk or juice or soda with your meals? I know it seems trifle, but tell me about it. What were your calories? Don't know? Send what you can. We will make what we can from what you know and get you going. But don't expect me to do all the work. I want you to learn, and educate, not become dependent. Then came the professor in college…. What were they thinking?

There wasn't a reason under the sun to open up any of those intimidating works of literature. BUT I would somehow find the time to read magazines... Or thumb through them for pictures... On occasion I would stumble upon some interesting stuff... Maybe read it… And that is what I meant about a short attention span. I too have one and I too would rather read a quick article than something ten pages long… Let alone several hundred pages long… Unless of course I am interested in it. And I thank you for that interest. I appreciate you so much that you can now receive additional copies of this book at a 50% discount by sending a check or money order with $3 to cover shipping and handling to our office.

You may join our monthly supplement refill club if they didn't come initially with this book for only $45 a month as well. To keep your life discreet and to save you from grocery store line embarrassment, we can provide for you half-gallon enema bags for $15 too. Just email me at the site for details.

One of my better known quotes: "If you are trying to get to Pittsburgh and drive past a sign saying Vancouver is 3 miles away, you're not heading in the right direction. You could keep going around the planet aimlessly and eventually only end up back where you started (drowning in an ocean of wasted effort) or you can turn around and use your new KNOW HOW."

Is there more? Certainly! Any of the below websites offer Don Lemmon's KNOW HOW (book two) that covers an introduction to gyms, home gyms, bodybuilding, my famous 4 Phases Of Training and Exercise Know How, 3 months of strict routines, 26 bonus workouts, my martial arts book, physique contest preparation secrets for dropping amazing amounts of body fat, boot camp training programs, pregnancy tips, recipes, menus, the personal training business guide, health questionnaires, fitness waivers for trainers, a chapter on natural health care and chiropractic, another on plastic surgery and sections for children, teens, baby boomers, seniors and male enhancement formulas. This book is now available at all Don Lemmon oriented websites and you will get it for 33% OFF by mentioning you have this book already in the order form's comment box!

Do not forget to look for our Log Book, Exercise Videos, the original Know How book on CD and our other specials when you visit these other fine Don Lemmon websites for information, bonuses, tools and things not offered in this book that may prove to be not only helpful but your missing link to success:

www.toneupyourbody.com - Our family oriented website portal.

www.donlemmonsknowhow.ca - For SPECIALS exclusive to Canada.

www.donlemmonsknowhow.com - To get more behind the eating and debunking of fads.

www.hardcoredrugfreebodybuilding.com - Our network head for bodybuilding.

www.yougottareadthis.com - My entertainment news magazine.

www.refusetofail.com - Self help taken to an all new level.

www.lemmonsoil.com - The now infamous essential oil blend.

www.perfectvitamin.com - The most potent multi nutrient around.

www.ultimateherbalformula.com - Healing herbs for all bodily needs.

www.glandularcomplex.com - Desiccated glands for hormone support.

www.completeproteinpowder.com - Finally, our own protein blend.

www.truthaboutexerciseandnutrition.com - Secrets not in this book which include an all in one new KNOW HOW book available there containing more menus, recipes, workouts, weight gain, bodybuilding, personal training business, martial arts, contest preparation and more....

For Don Lemmon's 8 current non-fitness related novels: www.frankensteincastle.com, www.itsjustanotherday.com, www.planetofthegods.com, www.gernblanston.com, www.whitediamondrockband.com, www.manmadevirus.com, www.vampirefilm.com, and www.mrlasvegasnevada.com

The first six stories are available all in one book. See any site for details.